The Enemy Within

One Vietnam Veteran Helps Others Cope with PTSD

By

Gregory A. Helle

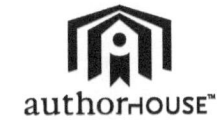

authorHOUSE™

1663 LIBERTY DRIVE, SUITE 200
BLOOMINGTON, INDIANA 47403
(800) 839-8640
WWW.AUTHORHOUSE.COM

First published by AuthorHouse 08/12/04

ISBN: 1-4184-1097-7 (sc)
ISBN: 1-4184-1098-5 (dj)

Library of Congress Control Number: 2004095479

Printed in the United States of America
Bloomington, Indiana

This book is printed on acid-free paper.

This book is dedicated to all those who

suffer from PTSD, regardless of the

source of their trauma(s).

and

to my family and friends

who have "walked" with me…

always by my side

as my God carried me.

and

to my very special friend

Joel Torres, USMC

Desert Storm

9/26/64 - 5/24/04

Your demons are now gone my friend

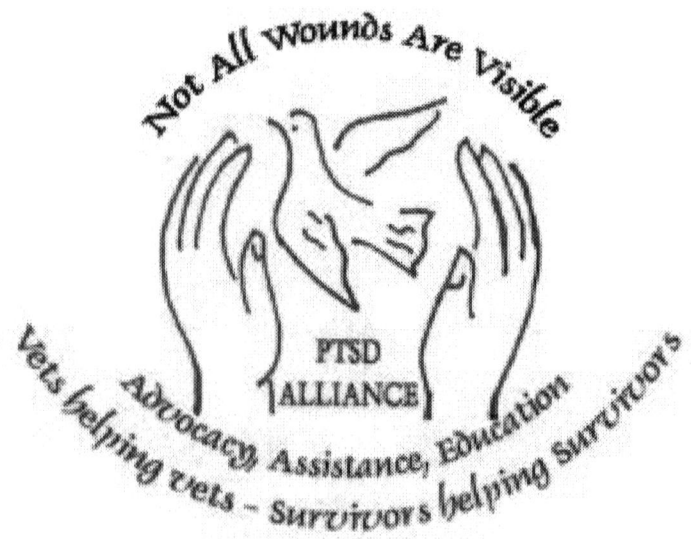

The author of this book has donated all rights and income to

PTSD Alliance

In hopes that all victims of PTSD find hope and peace

www.ptsd-alliance.org

Table of Contents

FORWARD: REFLECTIONS ON PTSD IN THE VIET NAM ERA VETERAN

I have never met anyone who was imprisoned in a concentration camp whose experience was so horrific that they could not remember it. Perhaps such people exist; I can not prove the negative by failing to discover anyone single one of them. What I have found in my clinical practice are hundreds of people who can not forget such experiences. In fact their inability to forget is so profound that it influences every aspect of their lives in negative ways. The natural history of exposure to horrific experiences such as combat, rape, natural disaster, or terrible accidents in which one fears for their life or witnesses the deaths of others is oftentimes to encode a special memory of these events which are lived in a world ruled by a distorted perception of the flow of time. These individuals can be catapulted back to the uncomfortable arousal and negative emotions associated with their original trauma by the slightest stimuli in their environment. An unusually hot and muggy day, a loud noise, the subtle smell of burning rubber in the air may erase the distance of 30 years and bring them back to re-live their previous horror as if it were going on that very day. These individuals die a thousand deaths and continuously carry that emotion with them. They suffer from Post Traumatic Stress Disorder (PTSD).Their inability to forget may also lead to the traumatic events being relived in dreams and their emotional dysregulation may manifest itself in many failed jobs and relationships. They simply can not get beyond the traumatic events in any normative way. There seems to never be enough "water having flowed under the bridge" to restore health nor cure their psychological wounds. They carry a pathological sense of doubt with them: am I safe, will all be well, can I survive?

Various studies have shown that among combat veterans of the Viet Nam War 15-30% show significant signs of PTSD 20 and 30 years after their service. Their suffering can take many different forms. Some continuously relive the emotions and memories of the traumatic events, existing in a chronic state of hypervigilence and hyper arousal. Others suffer from avoiding these memories and emotions though the abuse of alcohol and both recreational and prescription drugs. They live in a state of chronic numbness. Depression, anxiety and poor abilities to concentrate are also frequent pathological companions to PTSD.

Interestingly not all those exposed to significant trauma show the prolonged serious residua of PTSD. One of the most important challenges for Psychiatrists is to understand what might be the important elements that may lead a given individual to be more prone than another to develop the full syndrome of PTSD. It appears that the intensity of the initial response to the potentially traumatic event may be the most significant of all predictors for a longtime poor outcome to develop. If the initial trauma is so great, and their initial reaction to it so bad, many will be destined to relive it. Other predictors would include a past history of significant trauma, especially in childhood, and the preexistence of psychiatric disorders such as depression, manic-depression, panic, obsessive compulsive, and substance abuse disorders. If someone is not doing so well (Psychiatrically speaking) before serious trauma they will probably do much worse after experiencing horrific and life threatening events.

The treatment of PTSD can be divided into three realms: (1) helping the individual to come to terms with the original sensitizing traumatic event, (2) controlling the negative physiological reactions which endure long after the event and, most importantly, (3) helping the individual reintegrate into normal social, occupation and cultural contexts shedding an identification of himself as a victim of trauma.

With those returning from the Viet Nam War it was oftentimes most difficult for them to place their trauma and prolonged negative symptoms into a rational context which either made sense or offered comfort. For the most part they were not received in the USA with respect and military honors. If they were experiencing the symptoms of PTSD this was not a recognized diagnosis the way it is today. During those days medical care provided by The Veterans Administration hospitals was reserved for those who were judged to have their disabilities or disorders as "service connected". Yet many who came home from the WAR could not be seen by VA Physicians to have their conditions judged as service connected. This type of "Catch-22" was rampant at this time. Many went untreated and suffered without even an evaluation. They had a prominent and persistent disorder that did not even have a name. Their sacrifice and "wounds" were neither recognized nor honored. Many patients who were diagnosed were done so incorrectly as suffering from Schizophrenia or other psychiatric disorders. Patients were put on inappropriate medications frequently suffering from unwanted and severe side effects with no obvious clinical benefit. Many of these errors have been corrected by the VA Hospitals and by our society's reaction to soldiers returning to war. What have we learned? That some of the worst wounds can not be seen with the eye.

In my clinical experience many conditions which would be shorter lived negative states are prolonged through the misuse of alcohol, marijuana and prescription sedative drugs such as Valium, Xanax, and Ambien. Such medications not only cause states of numbing while the individual is acutely intoxicated but cause states of agitation and hyper arousal when an

Individual habituated to their use refrains from their consumption for short periods of time. Such individuals switch back and forth from intoxication to withdrawal. The first step in the judicious pharmacotherapy of PTSD patients should be their detoxification from such substances. Other medications may then prove useful for helping some of the physiological and cognitive difficulties encountered in PTSD. Among some of the most promising are the Selective Serotonin Reuptake Inhibitors (SSRIs) examples of these include Fluvoxamine, Fluoxetine and Paroxetine. These drugs are potent antidepressant, antianxiety and antiobsessional drugs. They may work directly in countering the "Pathological Doubt" encountered in PTSD helping suffers feel more secure that they will and can be safe.

As PTSD may be conceptualized as a disorder of remembering "too well" and not being able to easily forget, it is therapeutically important for a therapist to help someone, especially a soldier returning from battle, to reintegrate into a non military society. Therefore relationships, occupations and social activities that do not relate to the original trauma or its contexts are crucial for the Veteran with PTSD. Without doubt, sharing of experiences with other afflicted individuals can help PTSD sufferers feel that they are neither unique nor alone in their personal Hell. Yet all too often Veterans reinforce their PTSD by continuously wearing military-like clothing or insignias, associating only with other Veterans, or engaging in therapies that keep their focus only on their trauma without sufficient attention to developing a future disassociated from their war time experiences and identity.

These thoughts lead me to explore a very difficult conundrum in the treatment of war time PTSD: the role of the VA system of Hospitals and Clinics. No doubt well meaning individuals have set up a system that undoubtedly, besides doing much good, may inadvertently be prolonging the course of PTSD for many individuals. This is accomplished by providing financial incentives that may reinforce the sick role, promote too much focus on group association with similarly afflicted individuals, and give too much of a forum for the reinforcement of the self identity as a victim of war. This is a real conundrum as certainly those afflicted with PTSD are entitled to disability benefits, expert staffs of trained individuals are needed to assemble together in treatment centers and those similarly afflicted can provide shared comfort. This is a problem with no obvious solution.

In summary PTSD is a serious disease with serious consequences. The Viet Nam War survivors with PTSD offer unique challenges not oftentimes encountered in all wartime victims of trauma. As psychiatrists we need to study this condition so we can develop better treatments and better systems for the delivery of those therapies.

-- Boca Grande, Florida, 2004--

Joseph Deltito, MD

Clinical Professor of Psychiatry and Behavioral Science

New York Medical College

&

Consultant in Psychopharmacology, Greenwich, Connecticut

Jose Riefkohl, MD

Assistant Professor of Psychiatry

Emory University School of Medicine

Decatur, Georgia

THE CURSE

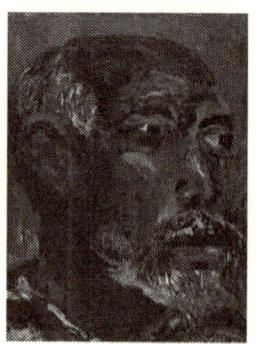

©Doug Yelman

Many years ago, I heard a rumor that soldiers who went to Vietnam were cursed. According to an ex-Buddhist priest, an entire sect of Vietnamese Buddhist monks spent years heaping specific curses upon all Americans who came to fight their country. These specific curses were:

1. That the American soldiers would become wandering men and women for the rest of their lives.

2. That they would never find peace.

3. That they would be angry men and women for the rest of their lives.

Another variation I have heard is that any soldier who comes to Vietnam will never leave.

Whether you believe in curses or not, there is much truth in these words for many of us. However, the same can be said of any war.

And the truth of these words is within many of us.

I sometimes feel sorry for myself, but mostly I hurt for my brothers and sisters who continue to fight, and to the new veterans and other victims who are faced with a hostile government and public who would rather just forget about war. We can't forget.

Greg Helle, 2004

INTRODUCTION

What would happen if there were a disease in this country that killed hundreds of thousands of people over the decades and left thousands more disabled? Suppose this disease drove many thousands of people to live cowering like hermits in the mountains and forests — or to bunker down, like me, in their own homes — just to survive. Such a devastating disease would make headlines. The American people would demand increased research on the causes in order to find a cure. They would develop foundations and strive to find ways to help victims lead productive and normal lives. Private benefactors and celebrities would hold lavish fund-raisers, and elected officials – and those who sought election to office – would wage very public campaigns to ensure that monies would be made available to find a cure. This would be of monumental importance in our society.

Such a disease does exist. It is called Post-Traumatic Stress Disorder (PTSD). Some may know it by the older terms of battle fatigue or shell shock. Most people, however, do not even know about this disease. Most who do know of it, or who know people with PTSD, assume it is a mental disease. It is seen merely as a weakness of the individual. But it is not a mental illness; it is the body's natural reaction to a horrific event. War is a common cause, and every war has its victims, on both sides. In addition to war, an individual can also develop PTSD through traumas in everyday life, such as rape (male and female) or other sexual assault; severe beating or physical assault; serious accident or injury; the sudden death of a family member or friend; witness to a killing or serious injury; natural disaster; and now, increasingly, terrorism.

None of us is immune.

There is a shorter-duration reaction to trauma called Post-Traumatic Stress Syndrome (PTSS), such as occurred to me after a car accident. However, there is some hope that with proper treatment at the syndrome level, it will not turn into a full-fledged disorder, and will have a lesser impact on the afflicted person's life. For this reason, early intervention *must* be a goal for the medical and psychological community. People who have PTSD want to lead normal lives; they want to hold down jobs, go to concerts and sporting events — but for too many, this is not a possibility. Perhaps it will be someday.

* * * * *

I am a Vietnam vet disabled with PTSD. I have PTSD from both combat and sexual traumas. I am not a Vietnam hero. I did not win medals for valor or wounds. I was not a grunt (an infantry soldier) so I did not see the worst the war had to offer. I went to war as a simple clerk, but that is not how my war developed. This is not an unusual story. Those who go to war do not have control over their lives or their destiny.

I served my country with pride, and have always considered myself a very strong patriot. I not only enlisted in the Army, I also volunteered for Vietnam. Right off the bat, I want the reader to know that I do not blame the military or the government for what has happened to me. My story is not about blame, but rather about recovery and healing. I was just a soldier who was in the wrong place at the wrong time. It has affected my life ever since. The war does not leave me, day or night. I am in a cage that I cannot escape. Medications help make the symptoms tolerable, but they only mask the symptoms. The emotions are always just below the surface.

In the pages of this book, you will get to know a boy who went off to war and was never the same after he came home. In many ways, I am not at home yet. It feels as if I left so much of myself in Vietnam and try as I might, I have never been able to bring it back. Some believe that a curse was put on men who went to 'Nam to fight, and as a result of that curse they would never be able to leave. In so many ways, this is true. That is why Vietnam veterans generally greet each other with the phrase, "Welcome Home." It sometimes seems to us that only other veterans can understand our inner feelings and our alienation from society.

* * * * *

Why would you want to read this book? There are several reasons. First of all, it is my hope that victims of all types of traumas, whether war-related or not, can find some comfort in these pages. If you are a victim of PTSD, you need to know that *there is hope for a better quality of life.* That is one of the core messages in this book. There is no cure for PTSD, but through medications and counseling, it is possible to exercise more control over the illness. But you must take the first step and be your own best advocate. You will hear me say this more than once. If you do not advocate for your own needs, it is unlikely that you will achieve your goals. I hope that some of the information in these pages will guide PTSD victims to seek the help they need.

I feel this book also has much to offer those who don't suffer from PTSD. It is the story of how a normal eighteen-year-old farm boy from a small town in Iowa went to war and, over thirty years later — at the age of fifty-two — became totally disabled with PTSD. It is my hope that this will help the public understand not only Vietnam vets, but also vets from all wars, as well as victims of other traumas such as I mentioned above.

There are so many fears that hold PTSD victims back from seeking help or even admitting to themselves that they need help. Even though all those around them can see the changes in the victim, it is hard for the victim to admit a problem. They see themselves as having some kind of mental illness. Victims are often paranoid and worry about what others are thinking or saying about them, even those people who have no inkling that there is a problem.

Sometimes, it can seem to the victim that everyone knows there is something wrong, and that everyone is talking about him or her.

The public must become aware of the disease and offer compassion rather than rebuke. Vietnam vets in particular have been a source of fear in the general public. The media has exacerbated this situation by its frequent portrayal of the vet as an imbalanced, rage-filled time bomb, just waiting for the circumstances that will set him off. Perhaps this has made for some "entertaining" movies, but it has also kept many veterans from seeking the help they needed, lest they find themselves branded with this ugliest of clichés. Even if the victim knows there is a problem, it is so difficult to ask for help, especially from a government that loaths to acknowledge the existence – much less, the debilitating nature – of this disorder. It should come as no surprise, then, that many victims do not want anyone to know about their "weakness."

Very simply, it is time to end the silence and the shame.

I realize that parts of this book will be difficult for the public to read. Reading a true account is not at all the same as watching violence on TV or at the movies. In these situations, the dead are not really dead and the cast is not really experiencing the events being portrayed. It is much more difficult when the dead stay dead, bodies are permanently mutilated, and the effects of the war will stay forever with those who experienced them. . The violence presented in modern entertainment should be taken as it is intended (though sometimes the level of violence in our "entertainment" is disturbing). True violence should be taken very seriously because it can happen to any one of us — at war or at home. Where a particularly violent movie can leave one unsettled for a day or so, actually living through a violent situation can produce a nightmare that lasts a lifetime.

I do not intend for this book to be political, nor do I want it to be an attack on the Department of Veteran Affairs (VA). However, I do believe that the policies enacted by the government have played a significant part in weaving the intricate web of my life.

Nor do I intend this to be a self-help book. I am not a psychiatric professional (even though I have been told that, for all practical purposes, I have, over the years, earned a Ph.D. in PTSD based on my recovery process). I am a victim, and I can only relay what I know from my own journey. If it helps even one victim, I will be blessed.

As I have mentioned, I fully realize that there are parts of this book that the public would rather not read. But it is essential that all Americans understand that the effect of war is not over when the end is declared. There are thousands of other men and women, from World War II all the way through the Iraqi wars, who are fighting the same fight I am. Our young men and women returning from Afghanistan and Iraq are already exhibiting signs of PTSD. There are also many thousands who suffer from PTSD due to non-war-related traumas, and these effects will continue for a lifetime. I wrote this book from the Vietnam viewpoint because that was my war, and it was where I experienced my traumas. But the truth is that I do not see many differences between the traumas I experienced and those that many people experience in everyday life. Americans simply cannot close their eyes to these victims.

So that is why I have chosen to tell my story. Although at fifty-three, some of the memories have faded, much remains. Many long-forgotten memories have come back to me in bits and pieces. I have done my best to recount them accurately and in chronological order. Yet because PTSD is woven into the very fabric of my being, it is difficult to isolate one event from another. Sometimes I feel the PTSD *is* me, because it rules so many aspects of my life.

I do not want you to feel sorry for me. I did not write this book to elicit pity, but to convey a message of hope for those like me. I am lucky, and God has endowed me with the ability to communicate in writing and speech for all those who cannot talk for themselves, for this is their story as much as it is my own. The only differences are within the details. I praise my God daily for the abilities he has given me, rather than blaming him for what has happened to me.

So, here we are… I invite you to walk with me through my life, and see with me the light beyond the shadow.

- Gregory A. Helle

CHAPTER ONE

HERE AND NOW

The statement I hear most when I discuss the effects of my disease is, "Just get over it." This statement is insensitive, and exposes the public's lack of understanding of post-traumatic stress disorder. If there were any way for PTSD victims to get over it, I would do just that, and so would

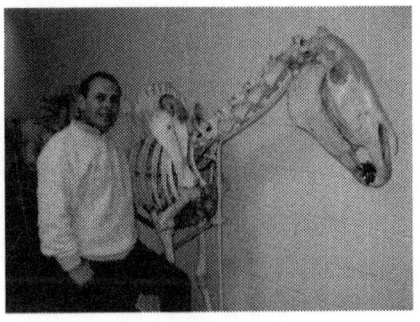

Greg when he was still working

every other victim. The face I put on for people usually appears normal, but the unfortunate reality is that there is no cure, and the "face" most people see is a manifestation of my desire to be "well." PTSD is like diabetes; it will be with me all my life. This is a reality that I must accept.

Is there hope? *Yes, there is hope.* My life is better than it has been in the past. I am maintaining my relationships and have even developed strong friendships with new people. Many of the simple things most people enjoy can be enjoyed by people with PTSD. Maybe I cannot participate in some of these seemingly uncomplicated activities with the same ease as normal people, but within those boundaries that I cannot change, I can enjoy life. All victims can learn to better cope with the disease and realize a better quality of life.

All victims of PTSD have boundaries, normally called triggers, which they may never be able to cross. Some of my triggers are crowds, noises or other activity in life that does not bother the normal individual but will cause fear, flashbacks, nightmares, etc. in me. There is only one person who can determine what these boundaries are — the individual with PTSD. This does not mean that these boundaries are permanent. Gradually, I am learning that I can overcome or learn to cope with these triggers. I may not be able to sit in a football stadium (yet), but I now am able to learn to shop in stores. Each step is small but significant.

I was recently driving through Colorado when a sign caught my eye: "Beware of falling rocks." Although I have driven by dozens of these signs, I was not hit by any rocks. That experience really struck me as if it were a personal warning to me. There are "falling rocks" out there that could knock me off the path I want to follow, returning me to where I was six years ago. I just need to keep my eyes open for them.

One of the major points I learned in my many hospitalizations and therapy sessions is that I must take "baby steps." That means I cannot expect to go from where I am to perfectly normal in one big step. This "giant-step" mentality has gotten me into a lot of trouble emotionally in the past. I remember coming home after ninety days in a VA hospital, honestly thinking I was cured. I learned later that this is sometimes called the "honeymoon phase." I did feel much better, but I also had been in a safe place where everything was controlled. It did not take long for real life to hit me in the face. Misreading my degree of recovery in this way was the cause of additional hospitalizations. PTSD victims must understand that every time they take two steps forward, they will probably take a step backward. But it is essential that we, as victims, take pride in accomplishments — no matter how small.

I am always aware that I may sometimes relapse to an old behavior. This is very discouraging for me, because I do not want to go back. Yet such relapses are not uncommon. It helps me to know that when I relapse, I am not alone. I know there are other victims who experience relapses. I also know that if I let myself believe that there is no hope, I will end up where I started. I refuse to do that. I know what types of behaviors I want, and a relapse is just another opportunity to work on myself. I am my most important project. I know that when my feelings are approaching a problem level I cannot handle by myself, I will seek out the help I need, even if that means more hospitalization.

There is always a catch (if you do not believe it, look at the VA. For all their strides in technology and their improvements in patient care, the VA system still reminds those of us who must deal with it of the meaning of the acronym SNAFU!). No professionals, family, or friends can make me – or any other PTSD victim – change. They can provide us with guidelines and support, but it is up to me to make the changes that will let me enjoy the things that are important in my life.

My answers may not be the same as those for other people with PTSD. This is not a cookie-cutter situation. Each person must find his or her own road.

I do know that I will never be the boy I was when I turned eighteen in 1968. That innocence disappeared before I turned nineteen. I accept the fact that the boy I remember is gone forever. I must also accept the fact that what might have been is gone. I have no clue what I might have been able to accomplish if I did not have PTSD. I am who I am. That is the reality of my world, and is something I can live with.

I realize that I must depend on medications to mask some of the problems and negative emotions I experience. Going it on my own is not an option. When I try to get along without my medications, I return to where I have been too often. I do not want to go back and re-experience that hell. This is my choice. The options available to me are greater if I maintain my medications.

I have a lot of fun talking about my drugs. The professionals hate it when I use the term "drugs," but I find some enjoyment in this. Some members of my family make jokes about some of the medications I take. I take a drug that is a mood stabilizer, which helps keep me from being physically aggressive. My son-in-law always asks if I have taken it before we go to the rifle range. I have the ability to look at my situation with a sense of humor. Feeling sorry for myself does not work.

I now have more good days than bad. However, the symptoms of PTSD have not disappeared, and I know that they never will disappear completely. Do not take this as negativity; it is just reality. I am thankful that, with appropriate medications and therapy, I have been able to exercise more control over the symptoms, and I am much more in control.

Like so many people with PTSD, I have my own little safe place, or "bunker," my office, located in the basement of my home. Even though I have a bunker, I force myself to go out somewhere in public at least once a day. I also leave my bunker when my wife is home. I know that isolation is a major problem for me and, therefore, I now know that I must do things that get me out into the real world, even if it is only for a short time.

Fear is a major factor. I know, at least on an intellectual level, that my fears are totally unfounded. In the last thirty years, I have not been personally attacked. Acknowledging that, I have usually been able to switch from carrying a gun to a pocketknife like the ones "normal" people carry – at least most of the time. Sometimes when I am alone at home, I do have my gun beside me. It is important to me to have guns even though they are usually locked up. The fear that pervades my life is a powerful force, motivating me to obtain more guns and ammunition to help me feel sure I can protect my family and myself.

A big part of the fear is not being able to watch everyone. I cannot cope with noise coming from multiple directions, and I cannot tolerate having anyone behind me. I always look for a table or booth in a restaurant that allows me to have maximum view of

5

everyone else, and I always know how to get out. Nevertheless, I can go to restaurants, though it sometimes takes a supreme effort on my part to do so.

I have been able to go to movies and other productions, even with people behind me. I find it necessary to know where those people are, and in these situations, there cannot be overwhelming crowd noise, lest my anxiety rise to a level I cannot tolerate. When I know that I will find myself in these situations, I take extra medications in case I cannot handle it. I do not want to embarrass my wife if I can help it. I am now able to run some errands for my wife, since I am at home all day. Sometimes, I can only go to one or two stores, leaving any others for the next day, but I can do it. The fear may never go away, but I have learned to control it or at least not let it control me most of the time. I am always hyper-vigilant in public, but I can accomplish small errands with the help of medications and my own personal resolve.

Another problem I have is with my appearance and personal hygiene. This is partially because of my memory problems – for instance, I will sometimes forget whether I have showered or shaved, or I'll neglect to get my hair cut. But it is also a defense mechanism. The less socially acceptable I look, the less people want anything to do with me. If people see that you look "different," they tend to leave you alone. Just as the public makes wide circles around the poor and the homeless, I would have them stay at a "safe" distance from me. Overcoming this tendency to hide behind a "dangerous" outward appearance is a major achievement in my efforts to deal with people.

There is a common conception that Vietnam veterans are crazy. When people know that you have PTSD, many become afraid. There seems to be an assumption that we are all "crazy" and that we will harm them in some way. This does help keep people away, but is so far from the truth. While the sick part of me appreciates the distance from others, the part that longs to be well feels the pain of that unspoken but obvious rejection very deeply. I have not physically harmed anyone since I was in 'Nam, and I do not think that I could harm anyone again. I do not need any additional nightmares.

The events that I experienced in Vietnam left me feeling like an outcast, since even talking about some of the things we saw and did is "taboo" in the eyes of society. I have found that my openness is a way for me to break down that wall between myself and the rest of the world.

Anger has been a major part of life since I got back, and there was not a big step from anger to rage. This made people feel the need to step lightly around me or, as my wife put it, "walk on egg shells" in my presence. While I have not physically hurt anyone since I left 'Nam, I would, on occasion, take my anger out on inanimate objects. I have been known to put my fist through walls and doors. Throwing things was common. When I could work at a regular job, my co-workers would often be afraid of me. However, I do thank my God that I never hit my wife or kids.

It has taken medication to reduce that anger level to the point that I have time to think about what is happening before it becomes a rage. I have not gotten to the rage point in a long time and usually, after I think about what has angered me, I find that there are ways to express that anger in a socially acceptable manner. I have learned to be assertive with my feelings, rather than bottling them up until they burst forth inappropriately.

Depression – which is really rage turned inward – has always been a problem since I came home, and became a serious problem when my world fell apart. I was locked up on several occasions when thoughts of suicide began to grow in my mind. A few times, I came very close to killing myself. I would actually inflict injuries, such as cutting myself, because the physical pain distracted me

from, and was so much easier to take than, the mental pain I felt. I know that for a long time, my wife fully expected to come home from work one day and find me dead. Medications have helped the depressions. They are not as deep as before, and do not last as long as they did before the medications. I have also learned that when I feel that depression building, I must distract myself by doing

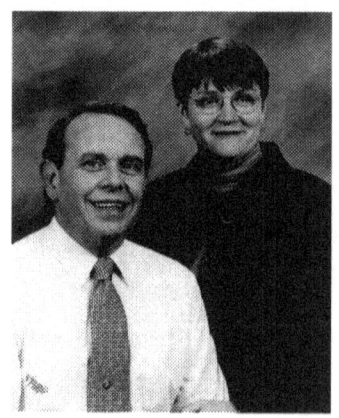

Alice and I

something different. It can be a very simple thing like a walk, but it can help me divert my attention from what is depressing me.

I still have occasional nightmares and flashbacks, but their power over me has been diminished. For a long time, a nightmare would often ruin my day. I would dwell on the nightmare repeatedly. This would detract from my effectiveness at work because I could not concentrate and was usually very exhausted. It got to the point where would go to bed afraid of sleeping, and would end up pacing

8

the house many nights, on constant alert for some unseen danger. Now with the help of medications, I can sleep most of the night. Sometimes I do wake up exhausted, but I am not bothered by the details of the night's dreams. Other times, my wife will awaken me from a nightmare, and I usually do not remember the dream. I have begun to realize that I do not have to dwell on events that happened so long ago, and I usually do not have to guard my house at night anymore.

One other problem is my lack of short-term memory. One of my therapists told me I had three things going against me – my age, my medications, and my PTSD. I just make jokes about it now. I keep a pad in my pocket to keep notes. If my wife wants me to do something during the day, we have a "honey do" list that I can refer to throughout the day. There is a good side to this. I can see a movie more than once and it seems new each time. This is something I cannot change so I might as well have fun with it. Sometimes laughing at yourself can help get you by.

I have a blessing that many victims of PTSD do not have. I have a very loving family and extended family. My wife has stuck with me for over thirty years. She has never wavered. I am not the man she thought she was marrying when she was nineteen. I asked her once why she did not leave me, and her reply was, "I married you for better or worse, and if this is the worst, I can handle it." For so many who returned from wars, their loved ones found themselves unable to deal with the changes, or had moved on in their absence. I can only imagine what it would have been like to come back from a war, damaged as I was, only to have someone I loved and counted on abandon me. Talk about something that would magnify an already monumental problem! My two children have stuck by me and have not felt that they have been harmed by my problems. They are not ashamed of what happened to me, have forgiven me when I have done some stupid things, and the best part is that they both still love me, even though I have changed.

My mother and my bothers and sisters have stuck by me as well, and provided an immense source of support as I struggled. One of my brothers calls me every week to check up on me. If he feels that I am down, I soon get calls from all my other brothers and sisters. When this happens, I know that he has called them and told them of his concerns. It would be impossible to describe how powerfully such things communicate to me the unwavering support I have. Sometimes, it might even feel like an intrusion, but I know how important that support has been, and am thankful beyond words for it.

I know that not every PTSD victim is so lucky. That is why I said that I am truly blessed. I have met many veterans in the hospitals, and I continue to work with veterans from around the country. Much of what I hear is the same, and most of what I am being told I can relate to, because I have been there myself.

Many veterans have a strong hatred or fear of the government, which extends to the VA. Many have no idea of how to file a claim, or they may not have the ability to communicate their problems. Many have been divorced, sometimes multiple times. Some have children who will not have anything to do with them. Some have been on illicit drugs for thirty years. There are differences between the veterans I have known, but there are many more similarities.

The worst problem is feeling alone. I initially believed that I was the only one who felt this way and the only one who could not handle my traumas. It sometimes seems this is a feeling that no one understands. Those who have seen psychiatrists feel that the only solution psychiatry can offer is medication. Those who see psychologists and social workers get the feeling that many of these professionals only know about PTSD from the textbooks they have read. There are many professionals out there who are ill-equipped to address the needs of people with PTSD. But I am assertive. I would not stop until I found people whom I could trust. They are out there as well; I have been with many who really care and can provide some real therapy, and will help you move on. I have also been in positions where the only course of action for me was to "fire" my counselor. I feel very strongly that the counselor's job is to help me cope with my problems. If that job is not being accomplished, I have every right to find someone who can meet my needs. I consult with some people in the local VA hospital that some of my friends cannot stand, and vice-versa. Personalities are different and so are psychiatrists, psychologists, and social workers. I insist on finding one with whom I am a good match.

The single most important thing is that I never give up on myself. Whatever happened to me is not my fault. I may never get back to where I was, but I can find a way to enjoy life.

I know that I can never go home again, and I am okay with that.

CHAPTER TWO

ALMOST HEAVEN

Growing up in Iowa was like growing up in heaven. It was a place where everyone cared. Iowa had – and still has – fewer people in the whole state than do most of the country's major cities. My memories of growing up there are strong and treasured. We were poor, but it felt like we had all the riches in the world.

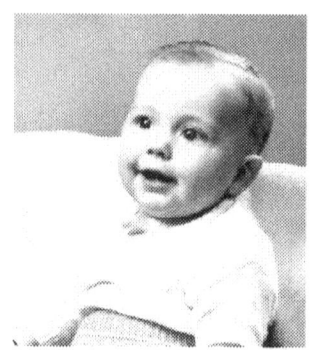

Greg when he was cute

My grandparents on my father's side emigrated from Norway, so I am second generation American. Maybe that is why people say I am stubborn. I do not think I am stubborn; I just have definite opinions on most things. We are still speculating about my mother's side, but I grew up more Norwegian than anything else, and still love Norwegian food, though at my age, I cannot handle all those calories anymore. There seemed to be one hard and fast rule for Norwegian food: it had to be white.

Maybe that is part of the reason why so many Norwegian kids, me included, were so fat.

I have few memories of my paternal grandfather. What I do remember is that he was very sick. I remember my grandmother as being a very large woman, very smart and loving. In addition, her cooking was fantastic, perhaps with the exception of her blood pudding. While she was brilliant in her preparation of everything else, I could just never warm up to the idea of pudding made from blood. In those days, however, no part of an animal was ever wasted, including things that no "normal," non-Norwegian person would consider eating.

My grandparents on my mother's side were a different story. I remember that while my grandfather always seemed to be happy to see us kids, my grandmother always seemed cold to us, so we would spend a lot of time doing other things in town instead of staying there. We were lucky that they lived in another small Iowa town called West Bend. The highlight of the town is a structure called the Grotto, a huge assembly of cement embedded with rocks and shells from all over the world. It was started by a local priest and has all the Stations of the Cross, along with other beautiful religious rooms. Although it was a religious structure, it was a playground for my younger brother, sister, and me.

I was a lucky child because I had three sets of grandparents. The third set was actually my great aunt and uncle, but they were always Grandma and Grandpa to all of us kids. Grandpa was always glad to have us around, and he would get down on the floor to play with us. Grandma was very loving, and one of the best cooks around. We always enjoyed spending time with them. Grandpa was an avid angler, but he died before I was old enough to go fishing with him. However, his hand-knotted fish keeper and some of his lures are hanging in my garage

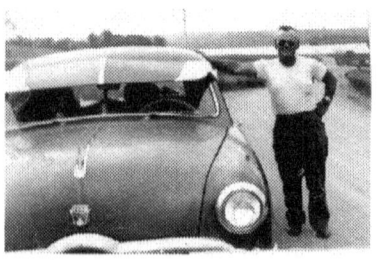

My dad, Albert Helle

to remind me of him. When Grandma died, I made sure to have some mementos of her too. I have a chest that was made from their first bed. It is nice to have something to treasure from those in my life who have passed on.

My parents went through the Great Depression, and experienced poverty in a way most of us – especially I – do not understand. I would listen to the stories they would tell, and could not imagine what it had to have been like. My mother's family had a hard time even putting food on the table, and were it not for a family who had a little more and would feed her after school, my mother would have often gone to bed hungry. Even after the Depression ended and the rest of the country seemed to be on a fast track to prosperity, life remained a struggle for both Mom and Dad.

My father, Albert, was a strong, stoic, hard-working man. I remember his arms being about as big as most people's thighs. He could never say that he loved any of us, but we all knew. There was never any doubt what Dad thought about his children. He once said he wouldn't take a million dollars for any of us kids, but wouldn't give a nickel for another.

My father had a very hard life. He was born and raised in North Dakota. I have seen a picture of the house where he grew up, and there was absolutely nothing around it. Save for the crops that grew in the warmer months and the snow that covered everything in the winter, it could have been a desert. During the Depression, he was a hobo, hopping the train from town to town looking for work. I really do not know how he ended up in Iowa, but he might

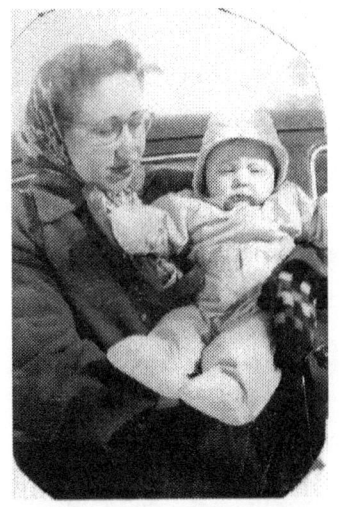

My Mom, Verna, and me

have been influenced by the fact that Iowa has a lot more trees and much less snow than North Dakota. He made his living as a sharecropper and dairy farmer, raising six kids on 160 acres of land. Nowadays, a person would be hard-pressed to support just himself on that same 160 acres.

My mother's life was not much better. She left her home when she was fourteen which was very common at the time. She spent much of her youth working for other people, washing clothes and keeping house. It was not much of a life for a young woman, but she, like so many others of that time, managed the best they could.

I am not sure how my dad and mom met. They were married on December 14, 1938, after dating only six weeks. They started out in a two-room house in Bode, Iowa, a little dot on the map. Things were very tough, not only during those early years, but throughout their lives. Dad would sometimes get the leftovers from a restaurant so they could eat.

The farm where I spent my first five and one-half years was outside Bradgate, Iowa. This was one of those towns whose name was almost bigger than the town itself. There was not much on the farm. There was no running water. We had a well, from which all the water we needed was pumped. Of course, no running water meant I was trained to use an outhouse. I often wondered, but have never asked my mother, whether it was tougher to toilet train children with an outhouse (they did stink) or modern facilities. When mom washed clothes – and there were four kids then – all the wash water and rinse water had to be hand carried in and out. They did not have a dryer at the time, so clothes were hung out in both summer and winter. Sometimes – especially in the winter – the clothes had to be hung inside the house to dry.

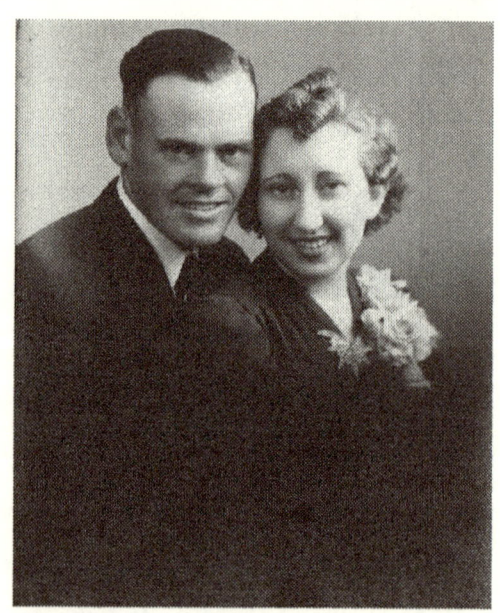

Albert & Verna Helle's wedding picture

I remember a story that our neighbor Earling told me so many times. The last time he told it, he was in his eighties and he still had tears in his eyes during the telling. As the story goes, I had been using the outhouse, and was trying to get my pants on as I came out the door. I saw Earling across the road, and as I waved at him, I accidentally dropped my pants. He said that was the only time in his life where someone greeted him with such enthusiasm that they exposed it all. Neighbors were very important, and there was a closeness (not to mention embarrassment!) that I have not felt since.

Life was so different back in the early 50s. The daily bath was not even a dream. During the week, we just washed up, usually in a basin of cold water outside. However, it was important to be clean for church, so baths were taken on Saturday nights. We had one bathtub in the middle of the kitchen floor. The water was carried in by buckets and heated on the stove. I do not remember how the order of baths was

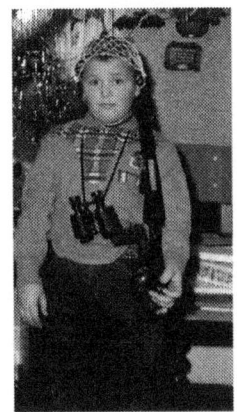

determined, but everyone in the family took a bath in the same water. While it would sometimes be heated up, the water was never changed. After everyone had bathed, the water was taken by hand outside, bucket by bucket.

Church was a very important part of my young life. We went to church in Bode, the town where my parents had begun their married life. I was baptized and married in this same church. The town of Bode was definitely a Norwegian town. A few miles up the road is an even smaller town, St. Joseph. Besides the Catholic Church, there is very little in this town, and the only reason you might guess it is a town at all is because of the church. As the story goes, the Catholics wanted to build their church in Bode, but the Norwegian Lutherans would not hear of it. The only church they would allow was their own Lutheran church. So the Catholics were forced to move down the road to build their church. Now, after all these years, there are two dying towns. Who knows what better fate might have befallen the two towns, had the Norwegians not been so stubborn.

Bradgate is now one of many dying towns in Iowa. Back then, however, it was the center of social activity. It seemed that everyone would go to town on Friday nights. I remember the five-cent Cokes; I think they were six-ounce bottles. There was also popcorn for the kids. We would watch a movie that was projected on the side of one of the downtown buildings. The seats were just planks across cement blocks, but it was a big thing to us. I am not sure what Mom and Dad did while we kids sat enthralled by the movie, but I imagine that Dad was with the other men, probably having a few beers, and Mom was somewhere with the other women. I will always remember

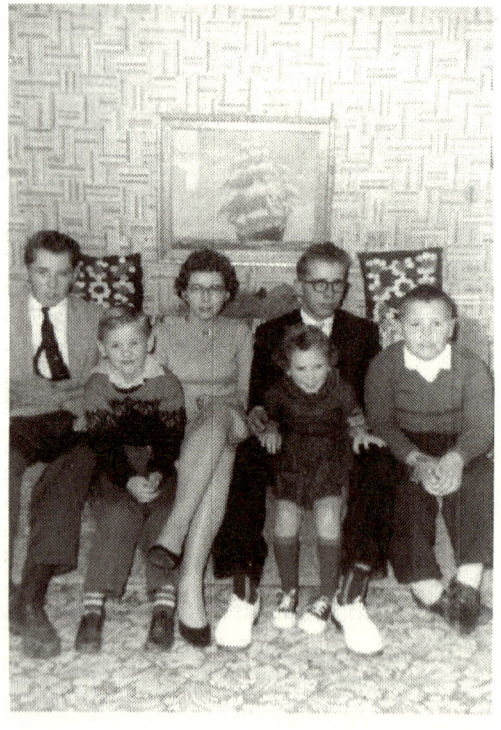

My siblings, left to right: Mick, Mark, Karen, Sue, Gene, and me.

that this kind of separation existed – and to a certain extent still exists – in my mother's life.

The Bradgate School sat high on a hill. If my memory serves me right, all grades were in the same building. Although I do not remember starting kindergarten there, I do remember that hill. In my young mind, it was the Matterhorn, Mt. Everest, and the best ski slopes in the world, all rolled into one. I still have cherished memories of winter afternoons spent careening down at a breakneck pace, clinging to my sled. I also remember the long climb back up. It seemed to take forever to reach the top, and a mere blink of the eye to hurtle back down. The school is no longer there, but when I drive by, the little kid inside me still gets the urge to fly down that hill on a sled.

We moved to a farm a couple of miles outside Dakota City while I was in kindergarten, probably around 1955. As had been the case with the farm in Bradgate, Dad did not own the land we lived on; he sharecropped again. I remember that the house we lived in was big and heated by coal. However, only the downstairs was heated. Our bedrooms were upstairs, and I think we had fifty pounds of blankets and quilts on us in the winter.

One of the major problems with coal heating, besides the fact that you had to keep shoveling the coal in and removing the cinders once it had burned, was that the chimney would get blocked. I remember many times waking up with a black face from the soot. Mom must have had a hell of a time cleaning up from that.

I remember Dad saying that he did not need a hired hand because he was raising his own. There were four of us boys, and Dad told us that if he gave us anything, he would give us the ability to work. He said if we were willing to work, we would never go hungry. My older brothers, however, keep telling me how lazy I was. They would get so upset with me that they would end up doing my chores. Maybe I was smart. When my older brothers eventually left home, I had to get more ambitious.

While they were still living at home, though, they taught me the chores with their own warped sense of humor. Once, when I was learning to load a wagon with bales of hay, they told me to start at the back and stack them up there first. Since the field was hilly, it was not long before the wagon was over-weighted in the back and would tip over; leaving the trailer, hay, and me sprawled on the ground. My brothers seemed to think this was extremely funny. I did not share their enjoyment at the time, but when I think about it now, I can't help but laugh, as well.

I had a brother who was three years younger than I. I was his protector, but he would have probably said that I was frequently more persecutor than protector. I taught him everything I knew. He was a real pain in the ass when he was young. For one thing, he would fall asleep anywhere – especially when he was supposed to be doing one of his chores. I had to get him out of trouble too many times. As it was my job to teach him all the "manly arts," I proudly taught him how to "water" most of the trees on the farm. Of course, then I had to teach him to stand on the stool when he was taking care of business indoors. Yes, we did have a real bathroom in that house, though there was only one, despite the size of the house and our family. We had white painted metal cabinets in the bathroom, and my mom told me she had to paint them at least once a year because of us boys.

One day the bathroom door was stuck, so naturally I put my shoulder to it. It came open quickly, but the basement door was just across a small hallway, and that door was open. I flew down to the basement without hitting a step, but landed head first in the coal

20

pile. When I came up, I was covered in blood. My Mom started to freak out, but my grandmother Helle was there. She got my head cleaned up and was able to stop the bleeding. Of course, no doctor was ever involved. I just hope I never go bald, because I must have one heck of scar on the top of my head. This stunt was forever after known as my Superman act.

To this day, my mother still feels bad that she was never able to buy us a swing set. She also wanted us to have a go-cart track, which also never happened. However, we never missed any of these things. We had a large pasture that provided endless hours of adventure for my siblings, my friends, and me. All it took was a good imagination. There was a river on the farm that we fished endlessly. I do not remember really catching anything good to eat, but the sheep-head and carp were fun to catch.

Despite the fact that we did not have money, the farm provided us with all the adventures we needed. We were surrounded by animals and naturally loved just about any kind of animal. At one time, we had a pet opossum. If you know anything about opossums, they are extremely ugly and really do not make good pets. We kept him in a shed and tried to tame him. I have no clue what opossums eat, but this one would not eat anything we offered. Despite all our loving care, the opossum didn't have a chance, and died on us within a couple of weeks. Naturally, we had to have a funeral for the poor thing. .

The farm had a cow pasture that seemed huge. I have no idea how many acres it was, but those hills were full of adventure. My brother and our friends would spend hours in that pasture having a tremendous time. One time we thought we were big enough to spend the night camping out there. We did not have fancy camping stuff, so Mom gave us the necessities for us to stay warm. We were having a lot of fun until the sun went down. Then there were the terrifying night sounds. I think it was an owl that really scared us. That is when we decided to go back to the house. Hiking back in the dark, however, we forgot that there was a big drop-off. We tumbled down that hill in the middle of the night and spent the rest of the night at the bottom of the ravine. We survived, but did not attempt it again for a while.

We also had a big hill in the pasture that was perfect for our winter games. We had several types of sleds and a four-man toboggan, and spent endless hours sliding down that hill, almost ending up in the river. One year, my older brothers built a ski jump using bales of hay and water. Although I did not ski, going over that jump was something I had to do. My little brother and I took the toboggan out and went over the jump. It was fantastic when we were flying through the air, but the landing was a little rough. I had let go of the toboggan and went tumbling head over heels down the hill. My brother held on, and just got a sore butt. I walked home, a little bloody from my landing. Mom fixed me up, needless to say. I had a sore arm, so she put an elastic bandage on it. After about a week, the arm still hurt. That is when she took me to a doctor. I do not believe my parents ever had health insurance. Anyway, they X-rayed the arm and it was broken. However, the week in the elastic bandage had allowed the bones to realign themselves, and all they had to do was put on a cast.

Our barn had a second floor that was called the haymow. This is where we stored much of the hay for our dairy cows. But leave it to us kids; it was another place of adventure. We would build forts all over the haymow with tunnels going all over. We would disappear for hours, especially in rainy weather and in the winter. When I think about the things we built in that haymow, I often wonder why none of our structures fell in on us. Some of them were so complex that it would have been hard to find us if they had tumbled down on us.

Like most barns, we had an overabundance of pigeons and rats. We would take our BB guns into the attic with us and do a considerable amount of bird hunting. I was a pretty good shot with that old BB gun, and had a pretty debilitating effect on the bird population. The rats would mainly be found in the cow feed room. They were pretty clever, but no match for us. We had an old .410 shotgun rigged up in the doorway of the feed bin, and every time we walked by, we would just sight down the gun and see if there were any rats. If I saw one, I would shoot it. With the shotgun, there was never any clean up. The rat just became extra protein in the feed.

As a result of our move, I had to finish kindergarten in Dakota City. Since we lived on a farm, we had to catch the bus to school, and I can remember many mornings, sitting on the bus and picking manure out of my shoes. When I told this story to my children, it seemed to gross them out. However, most people on the bus were doing the same thing. Kindergarten in Dakota City is where I met a boy who became – and remains to this day – my best friend. Our lives have way too many similarities. I remained in Dakota City through the sixth grade. (This was as far as either of my parents went in school.)

I have very few memories of my grade school days. I think I probably did fine, but school was never my favorite place. I do remember being caught cheating on a very simple word during a spelling test in the third grade, but I cannot remember what my punishment was. I also remember a girl named Beth – my first crush – in the fifth grade. I still have a picture of her somewhere with my mementos. She was not particularly interested in me, but I thought I was in love.

I went to junior high in Humboldt. I half-heartedly went out for football and track, but soon figured out that I didn't belong in any sport that required running. I did, however, like the shot put and discus. I eventually learned that I was not much of an athlete. At about that time, I started dating a girl named Linda, the daughter of a cop who really didn't like me very much. I did not drive at the time, so we would meet at the local dance hall. Linda was the first girl I ever kissed; but that's as far as it went. At that point in my life, I had no clue about anything else that I was supposed to do.

There was something about our farm that attracted many of the kids from Dakota City. We always seemed to have a group of our friends around. We put them to work, of course, and they seemed to love the chores. More than once, my dad would start a water fight, and pure pandemonium would break loose. I still remember one of my brothers chasing a friend down the road with a bucket of water. Dad wouldn't discriminate when he started one of these water fights. Everyone within range knew they were going to get wet, so there was no reason not to participate. Those water fights lasted well into my forties, so my children were exposed to a little of the fun I had as a kid.

One of my most powerful memories was of one day when my dad was teaching me to run the tractor and bailer. This was my first time doing this. We were stopped because of some kind of problem with the bailer. I was on the tractor and my Dad was working on the bailer. All of sudden I saw him wrapping a red handkerchief around his hand. He came up to the tractor, shut it off, and said we needed to walk home. It was about a mile home. We walked and talked. I had no idea what was wrong but figured we needed some kind of part for the bailer. When we got home, he told me to stay there and he drove off in the car.

It was a long time before they told me the truth. A bailer has forks that pack the hay into a bale. One of the forks caught his watch and went through his hand, leaving less than an inch of flesh holding his fingers to his hand. Even though he must have been in agony, he never showed any pain. The doctors managed to put his hand back together with a lot of wire, and he had about 80% use of the hand after it all healed.

It is said that the best things can come about as a result of a tragedy, and Dad's accident proved how true the saying is. Dad was laid up for a long time, and we kids could not do all the fieldwork. Without asking, all the neighbors from miles around came to our little farm and harvested the corn and beans for us. It did not take them long, since all of them had their own equipment working in the fields. The neighbors really saved our crops that year, but more important than that, they really taught my siblings and me the true meaning of friendship. The memory of their generosity has always touched my heart.

As a farm boy, I was involved with 4-H, which is a youth group that taught us about all the facets of farming. For my 4-H project, Dad gave me a calf. I called her Flicka, after the horse in a movie I had seen. Flicka was my pet, as well as my 4-H project. She had broken her tail at some time, so there was a knot at the top of tail where it healed. Although she was "defective," I was so proud to show her at the county fair. We sold her when we had to leave the farm, and it was like selling a friend.

A dairy farm was very labor intensive. We were up every day at 5:00 AM to milk the cows. After that was over, we had crops to maintain. That was back in the time when we walked the length of each row of our soybean fields, cutting out weeds by hand. I remember one field that was a mile long. I have no clue how many miles we would walk in a day, but I know that I hated that field when dad planted beans. We also raised a lot of hay to feed the cows. There were several crops a year, so I got very strong throwing around those 100-pound bales. My brothers and I would have contests to see how many bales we could get on one rack, then hold our breath, hoping it would stay together until we got it home. In the evenings, the cows needed to be milked again.

Since the cows needed to be tended every day, and wouldn't listen to any excuses, it made it hard to get away for vacations, but we would take a few day trips. I remember once going across the bridge to Wisconsin and thinking it was such a great thing to be in another state. The only real vacation I remember was a few days in the Black Hills of South Dakota. We camped under a tent that was nothing more than a tarp strung across a rope tied between two trees. Somewhere on the way, we passed an alabaster hill. I remember the fun of climbing that small hill, but I have never been able to find it again. Even though that vacation was only a few days long, it was great to be so far away from home.

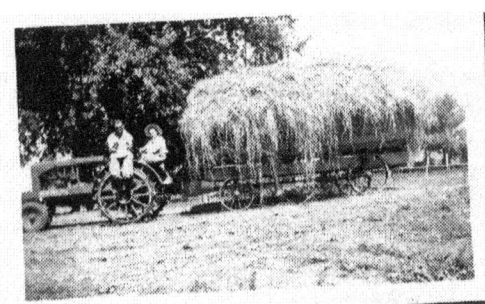

My dad early in his farming career

I cannot imagine growing up anywhere but on a farm. The stories I have told do not begin to portray the real essence of farm life. The entire community helped raise the kids. Neighbors would give the shirt off their backs to help you. I remember neighbors and friends always getting together, especially on a Sunday afternoon, just to talk and enjoy each other's company. This was not formal and much of the time, it was just a spur of the moment thing. As kids, we had so many adventures on each other's farm. This was the large community I grew up in. For the most part, it is a world that does not exist today.

When I was fourteen, the owner of the land sold the farm. My father had no choice but to sell his animals and equipment and move the family into town. After everything was settled, all he had to show for his thirty years of farming was enough to make a down payment on a four thousand dollar house. We were forced to leave the world of farming. Dad started working in a factory and Mom started to clean houses to make ends meet.

After a lifetime of hard work, Dad and Mom were left with nothing but memories.

CHAPTER THREE

THE "WRONG SIDE OF THE TRACKS" –THE YOUNG MAN COMES OF AGE

There are two towns adjacent to each other in northern Iowa: Dakota City and Humboldt, separated by railroad tracks. I was literally from the wrong side of the tracks, living in Dakota City, the poorer of the two communities. The social pecking order in school was based, for the most part, upon which side of the tracks a kid came from. While the "elite" were from Humboldt; there were also parts of Humboldt that were poor like Dakota City.

Like many rural kids whose families move into a more "urban" setting, I went through a kind of culture shock when we moved to town. I was accustomed to getting up early in the morning to do my chores before school, but that was no longer necessary. There were a few chores I had to perform around the house, but they did not take much time to complete. That left me with a lot time to do whatever I wanted, which sometimes was not a good thing.

Wrestling was the only sport that I went out for in high school. I had learned in junior high that any sport requiring running did not work well for me. My legs were way too short to be a runner of any kind, so my career in track and field really was not going anywhere. On the other hand, short legs were an asset in wrestling. I was a strong farm boy and did not mind mixing it up some. I was good – not a super star, but good. Unfortunately, my wrestling career died when I discovered girls. I remember warming up for a match doing pushups with a cheerleader on my back– great for impressing the girls, but not for my wrestling career.

My biggest problem in high school was my suddenly raging hormones. I was not a bad looking kid (age has now taken its toll), and finding girls – most from the wrong side of the tracks – was no problem. I would date several girls at the same time, even going steady with more than one. As you can imagine, school was the least of my concerns. I had more important things to do with my time.

When I was 15 or 16, I got a job at the local creamery (milk processing plant). I worked from 5 AM until it was time to go to school, and then returned after school to work a few more hours. At first, I spent all my money on clothes, but during the last two years of high school, I had a different car every six months. Back then, I could get a decent car for less than $500. Even though I was able to find ways to earn the money to support my car obsession, my poor dad had to co-sign many loans for me.

My favorite car was a 1957 Ford hardtop. It was a beautiful black car, great for getting the girls. In addition, it had a lot of "guts."

I remember once having the speedometer buried at 120 and still going higher. Every window in the car was shaking, and my tires were close to being bald, but at this time of my life, I was invincible. This poor car met its end when I turned off a blacktop onto gravel doing about sixty, lost control, and took a tour of the ditch. I was able to drive out, but all the Bondo™ that filled the holes in the body fell out, leaving my car looking like it had been through a war zone. It was clearly time for another car.

Having a car gave me a wonderful freedom. I could go just about anywhere, anytime I wanted. Drag racing was a big thing for me. I was, and still am, a pretty inept mechanic, so my car usually didn't run well enough to win. The thrill of racing was exhilarating, nonetheless. We would head down the road, side by side as fast as we could, often on bald tires. The cops wanted to catch us, but there were so many blacktop roads to drag on that their chances of being in the right place at the right time to catch us were pretty slim. They never did catch us dragging.

Although I had a tendency to wreck my cars, I had an old Buick that I just couldn't destroy. I hated that car. It was more like a tank than a car. It could only lay rubber in reverse, which looked somewhat ridiculous. No matter what I tried, that damn car kept going. This was the first car I owned that had some residual value when I traded it in.

A daily ritual I had was to pick up a friend who lived three blocks from me. In that short distance, I would get my car up to seventy miles per hour, hit the brakes, and do a 360-degree spin, leaving me facing back toward my house. I enjoyed the speed and the thrill of sliding on that gravel road. One day however, there was another car at the first intersection, with a mother and three children inside. I was already going too fast to stop, and broadsided that car. I was extremely lucky that no one in either car was hurt, but both cars were totaled. That night, my parents made me call the people I hit to check on them. That was an extremely difficult call to make. I lost my license for a while, which slowed me down and, for the most part, made me much more cognizant of my driving habits.

When I wasn't drag racing or wrecking my cars, I found another diversion: playing hooky from school. One of my girlfriends could copy my mother's writing exactly, so I had a handful of excuses for being absent from school. Several of my friends and I would frequently skip school and go on a road trips. Everything was going exactly as planned until one day we ran into one of our teachers in a town several miles away from Humboldt. Our game was over.

When I got home that night, my father already knew. Needless to say, he was very upset with me, and all I could get out during our "conversation" was "Yes Sir." The next day, the principal expelled all of us for three days. However, he did not allow all of us to have the same three days off. The punishment seemed odd, since I really did not want to be in school in the first place. I had achieved a reputation as one of the bad boys. My two older brothers had left me a challenge to live up to their reputations, and I think I was doing a pretty good job of it.

I enjoyed shooting in high school, and belonged to the local rifle and pistol club. My dad had taught me to hunt with a single shot .22 while we were on the farm. With that rifle, after taking a shot,

I had to eject the round and physically put the next round into the chamber. Dad always told me that if I needed the second shot, I was not really hunting. The rifle and pistol club owned several old M-1's that we would use for target practice, and I had several guns of my own. I remember shooting pennies that I had placed in trees to impress my girls. I am not sure if it did impress them, but I was a very good shot, even with open sights. At that time, I had no clue about scopes.

One Saturday night, the worst thing that can happen to a 16-year-old happened: I did not have a date. In desperation, I went to Bode and showed up at the home of some people I knew who had a cabin on Spirit Lake, right beside my best friend's grandfather's cabin. I had been going to Spirit Lake for years with my friend. I had known his neighbor Alice for a long time, but had never been particularly interested in her. That night, however, I just showed up at their door and asked if I could take Alice to the movie in town. That was back in the days when there was actually a theater in Bode. Alice was 15 at the time, and was not allowed to date until she was 16. I think they allowed me to take her since they knew me (*big* mistake!). We went to the movie, and then stopped by to visit my grandmother, and I got Alice home early.

There was something very different about Alice. She was smarter than the other girls I was dating, and her family was much like my own. So we continued to date. The second date was not as puritan as the first. I took her to one of my favorite places down by the river, where we could watch the deer. I was still dating two other girls at the time, and since Alice had to be home at 11 PM, I would sometimes have a second date on the same night. It was becoming a hard juggling act, since I had to be at work at 5:00 AM. It was not long until Alice was the only one I was dating.

Even though I was no longer on the wrestling team, I still enjoyed mixing it up. There were rivalries among most of the "big" towns around Humboldt. We would have fun going to other towns and having a good fight; I tell my kids that I was a gang member when I was young. Fortunately, no one really got seriously hurt. We had one guy who was a big as a house. We would go to Fort Dodge, the biggest town around, where another friend and I would cruise the strip looking for a fight. With Humboldt County license plates, that was not too hard. We would head to a park with our huge friend hunkered down in the backseat. We would instigate a fight, and then he would get out and finish it while we watched the fun. We didn't even have to get our hands dirty.

One day Alice and I were in a restaurant in Humboldt and some guys from another small town came in. They knew me and I knew them because we had gotten into a fight once before. They were harassing me, so I told Alice I needed to go outside with these guys for a while. She was not happy because there were several of them and only one of me. I told her it did not matter. If they beat me up, the whole bunch of us would be in their town soon and kick their butts. Alice just looked at me and said that if I went out there she would be gone when I got back. While I might have been overdosing on hormones and teenage invincibility, there was a limit (somewhere) to my stupidity, and I learned my lesson that night. That was the last time I fought in high school.

I did graduate from high school, much closer to the bottom of my class than the top. I remember getting the diploma and immediately opening it up to make sure it was signed. I was very relieved. That night, my family had invited many friends to our house. I had taken my best friend home, and was headed home myself when, about a block from my house, I saw that they were digging a ditch across the

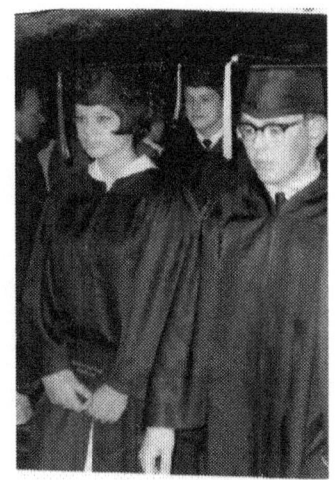

road for water or sewer. The ditch was not very wide, and the Chevy I had at the time was fast. In my mind, I knew that if I got my speed up, I could jump that ditch. Wrong. The front wheels went down the ditch and the car came to an abrupt – and very noisy – halt. That little event broke my front axle. As I got out of my car, I could see Dad and most of his male friends in our front yard watching my stunt. That one took a long time to live down.

Halloween in small town Iowa was a lot of fun back then. On most Halloweens, everything in town that was not tied down ended up on Main Street. The cops, figuring we were only kids letting off some harmless steam, just watched us. Nothing was hurt; we just had fun. Every year, someone would bring in a tractor so we could drag the nearby outhouses to the main street too. Several residents tried to find ways of keeping their outhouses secure, but the more they tried, the more determined we became, and the outhouses became a yearly fixture on Main Street. Usually, some of our dads would come in the next day to clean it all up.

Back then, "trick or treat" had a very different meaning. Our take on that term was that if you did not give us a treat we would play a trick on you. Some of the tricks we pulled were simple and harmless, like soaping the windows of the house. The nastier people would get the rotten tomato or rotten egg treatment on their house. The *real* nasty ones would get the big one: we would fill gunnysacks full of fresh manure, place the sack on their front step, set it on fire – and then we would ring the doorbell and run. Of course, we stayed close enough to watch them stomp out the fire, only to be covered in manure. I know it seems nasty now, but it sure was a lot of fun at the time.

Small town kids seemed to become sexual at a very young age, partly because there was not much else to do. Of course, there were always some kids who "had to get married," but I guess I was just luckier or smarter than they were. Looking back, I'd have to admit that it was probably the former, rather than the latter.

It is very important to understand the values of small town Iowa. There were three major values in life: God, Country, and Family. That did not mean we were angels, though it should be noted that when I graduated from high school, I had already made plans to go into the ministry.

My war really started in 1968 when my high school counselor told me that the only place I would make it was in the Army. I was not a standout – at least, not scholastically – in high school. It was not until my senior year that I actually started taking school seriously, due in large part to the fact that I was dating a young woman who could get straight A's without even trying. I fell in love with this young woman and changed my ways. However, the counselor, who had long been familiar with my behavior, could not see anything worth saving in me.

My goal was to join the Marines. They were the toughest guys around. However, a friend of mine who lived on a farm about mile from ours and was a year older joined the Marines. He was a chubby kid but when he returned home from basic there was no fat on him and that dress uniform was so sharp. Then and there I knew I had to go to the marines. After his leave, he was sent to Vietnam. On his first mission a bullet caught him under his chin. The next thing I knew I was attending his funeral. I did have a change of heart about becoming a marine.

When I was seventeen, I enlisted in the Army on the delayed entry program. This allowed me to finish high school before going on active service. I had been watching the war on TV, and knew it was where I needed to be. I knew nothing of the politics of the war. I just knew that I had an obligation to serve my country whenever and wherever it needed me. Now was such a time. When you enlist in the Army they allow you to pick where you want to go, and I chose Vietnam.

I was supposed to go on active duty in June 1968, but the Army determined that I could not go because of a thyroid problem (which I don't think I ever had). And then, wonder of wonders, the Army lost my records, leaving me free and clear. I did not have to go, and had a clear conscience because I had honestly tried to serve my county. I had been hearing about all those guys running to Canada to avoid going to war, but I had volunteered to go to war, had done my duty to my country.

In the summer of 1968, I went to Des Moines – the "big" city in Iowa – primarily to get away from my small hometown. I found a job in an Army surplus store and lived at the YMCA. For all practical purposes, I was broke. I always ate in a small diner close to the "Y", my daily menu rarely changing from a bowl of cereal in the morning, tomato soup for lunch, and a hamburger for dinner. Besides the rent, that was all I could afford. Even though I was only getting by, there was no way I was going to tell anyone at home. I was now a man, making it on my own in the "big city."

In the fall of 1968, I started going to a business trade school in Des Moines, the American Institute of Business. During my last year in high school, I had taken the business curriculum. Although I had gotten through my first three years of high school by the skin of my teeth, I was named "student of the year" for the business curriculum, so it made sense for me to go to business school. I never really thought about college. No one in my family had ever gone to college, and I was not sure that was the route for me.

I found an apartment on Nineteenth Street in Des Moines – not a very safe part of town. My roommates were also going to the same school as I, the American Institute of Business. Although I was doing well in school, my roommates introduced me to drinking and drugs – nothing major, because we were all broke. I always pitied the girlfriend of one of my roommates, because we really did nothing to keep the apartment clean. She would find dishes in the sink with mold on them. Bless her; she would spend all day cleaning up the mess, knowing it would soon be back the way it was. My roommates were city boys, so there were many differences between us. Even though I tried to fit in, I was never comfortable with that party crowd. I never got used to the part of town I lived in, either. Here again, I never told anyone at home, because I was a man and I was going to make it. John Wayne, all the way.

It was not long until the Army found my records (which had ended up in Maine), and they decided that I was in good enough health to go to 'Nam. At that time, I really think that having the ability to breathe and walk were the only required qualifications for duty. I withdrew from school and used the refund of my tuition to buy my girl an engagement ring. That somehow seemed more important than paying my school loan back immediately. I had a little time at home before I was to be put on a bus for basic training, and I spent as much time as possible with Alice, who was a senior at that time (I was 18, and she was 17). I occupied myself with painting my parents' house while she was in school.

In early October, I gave Alice the engagement ring outside during a high school dance. Later, we went to her folks' place. We were very nervous. We knew her parents liked me, but enough to let their daughter marry me? After straining to keep the small talk flowing for awhile, her dad started to go upstairs to bed. We called him back down, telling him we had something he needed to hear, and we wanted him to hear it from us. Alice showed him her engagement ring, and her dad just sat down and took off his shoes, muttering "Thank God that is all it is." We promised that it would be many years before we got married.

I knew I had the military ahead of me for three years, at least a year of that in Vietnam. I did not think it would be right to get married until I could stay at home. Little did I know that although I would be coming home, a very big part of me would be lost in the jungles and rice paddies. I would live, but my peace of mind – and my innocence – would die.

CHAPTER FOUR

TO HELL AND (PARTWAY) BACK: THE MILITARY

Talking about the war is very difficult for me. Libraries have bookshelves full of Vietnam stories, which I find myself both drawn to read, yet repulsed by at the same time. There are stories of those who had to endure much more than I did, and I realize that I was lucky in so many ways. Nevertheless, the effects that my experiences had on me are the same as all those who saw the worst of the combat. I am not apologizing for my service in 'Nam. I did what my country asked of me, and I am proud that I served.

I have not tried to tell you every story that I could tell to this point. I just want you to understand what it is like to go from a small town in Iowa to war.

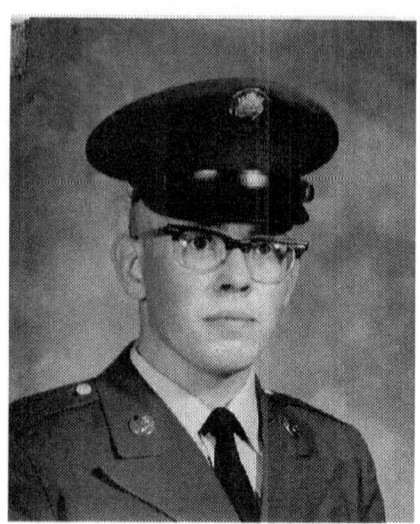

My official picture

METAMORPHOSIS: TURNING A COUNTRY BOY INTO A SOLDIER

In October 1969, I left for basic training at Fort Polk, Louisiana. This post —affectionately known as the "armpit of the Army" —is down in the middle of Louisiana, where no respectable man would want to go. But for the next three years, I had very little choice in my life. I belonged to the Army, and they made sure we understood the ownership rights.

When I got off the bus, I immediately knew this was not Iowa. We were forced into a rough formation and were called about every name in the book. The drill instructor would get inches from my face and tell me what kind of "piece of shit" I was, and how my "mommy was not here to protect me anymore." After growing up in the safety of my small hometown, I was surely not accustomed to that kind of irreverent treatment. They ran us through the barbershop, if you can call it that. In a few seconds, I was left with no hair. I had worked hard to have a full head of hair. They then ran me through supply, where I was issued my uniforms. There was no concern for the fit of the uniform. They just glanced at me and threw the uniforms at me. It was all so strange. Nothing in my youth had prepared me for this experience.

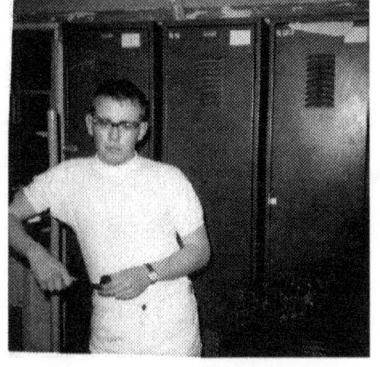

Me in Basic Training

Then in a rough formation, they led us to our barracks. I had no voice in the decision of which bunk I had or whether I was on top or bottom. The drill sergeant made sure that no questions were asked. Each of us had a locker and footlocker. We were given very definite instructions on how all of our belongings needed to be displayed in the lockers. We soon learned that it was more important to keep all our belongings ready for inspection, rather than using them. Like everybody else, I soon went to the PX and purchased additional items that were not to be used, but left in perfect condition, ready for display. Even our socks had to be rolled in a very specific way. If you looked at the top tray of the footlocker, it was always perfect. I would never touch this clothing, because it was only for inspections. I kept the clothes I wore separately.

Everyone needed to buy additional uniforms. When I fell out for morning reveille, it was expected that there would be a crease down the middle of my pants and a definite crease on the arms of my shirt. When uniforms were taken to the laundry, I had to ask for heavy starch, which meant that they came back almost as hard as a rock. I honestly think that they would have stood up by themselves. It was difficult to get my arms and legs into the uniform, and. I was very careful putting it on, because I did not want to ruin the look. The boots were also very important. I soon learned to spit shine the shoes until they were so shiny that I could see myself in them, no matter how much mud I had crawled through the previous day. The same went for the brass buttons on our uniforms. We went through gallons of Brasso™. The standards were so high that somebody always failed to meet them, which inevitably resulted in duty that was far from glamorous.

Even the lavatory brought a shock to me. The communal showers and the row of urinals were something I had experienced before, being a common occurrence in most school locker rooms. What shocked me was the row of open toilets, lacking anything resembling partitions between them. There was absolutely no privacy. I just had to sit there and do my business – including some things that were meant to be done in private – in front of God and everyone. This was one part of basic training that I found to be very humiliating, but there were more surprises to come.

Harassment seemed to be a major part of basic. They would wake us up at various times of the night for inspections or a march to nowhere in particular, for no discernable reason. The drill instructors were always on our case, and had no trouble swearing at us and telling us what our mothers were like. This was supposedly to take away our individuality and make us a fighting unit. I was determined not to let this mindset sink in for me. I would naturally help and cover

44

for my friends or anyone in our training platoon, but I convinced myself that this was due more to my hatred for the drill instructors than to any loss of individuality.

One of my worst memories from basic happened every morning. Before breakfast, they took us out for a nice little two-mile run. Not that two miles is that long, but I was endowed with very short legs. I am five foot seven with a twenty-nine inch inseam. My brother in law is six foot four. When we sit together, we are the same height. That tells you how short my legs were. Anyway, try as I might, I was always one of the last to complete the two miles, and one of the last in the mess hall. This usually meant that my food was colder than normal, and that some of the more palatable entrees were gone. Of course, this gave the drill instructor reason to harass me all the more.

The length of my legs also got me in trouble when we were marching. I swear that they would put the longest legged men at the front of the column. For every step they took, I had to take two. Try as I might, I could never stay in step with them. And this was just another reason for the drill instructors to jump my case. Being a strong Iowa farm boy, I wanted so badly to shut them up. Luckily, I held my temper.

There was one drill instructor that I hated the most. He was a squirrelly little man. He was a private first class, but you could tell from his uniform that at some time he had held a much higher rank. I figured that he was just a bastard, and that this was the only place the Army could put him. Here, at least, he could be a bastard without ever getting into trouble. Two months after basic,

I outranked him, and I really wanted to go back and give him the same kind of grief he had given me. To this day, when I see people who look something like him (and one was my boss for a while), I get the urge to kick the shit out of them. Logically, I know these are different people (mainly because they are a lot smarter), but I still hold a grudge to this day. It is amazing to me that I can still hate a person after all these years, even when I've convinced myself that he was just doing his job. Maybe it was because he enjoyed it so much.

Weapons' training was an interesting ordeal. For beginners, the instructors were fanatical in their insistence that we call them weapons, rather than guns. If a soldier used the term "gun," he would have to stand in front of everyone with his weapon and alternately point at the weapon and his crotch, saying, "This is my weapon (rifle), this is my gun (crotch), this is for fighting (rifle), and this is for fun (crotch)." I had to perform that ritual more than once, but I still call them guns.

The penalties for screwing up varied. The worst one I had was a time that we were out on the rifle range. We shot in groups, and when it was not our turn for shooting the guns, we kept them in a rack. The instructors were in rare form that day, constantly in my face. The harassment they were giving me was so intense that there was not even time for me to form an independent thought. When it was time to board the buses back to the barracks, I was apparently not moving fast enough, and instructors were screaming at me that I was the biggest screw-up in the platoon. When we arrived back at the barracks, I was quickly told that I had *really* screwed up, as I had left my weapon at the range. This was one of the supreme mistakes a trainee could make. Of course, there had to be punishment, and they came up with a good one. I spent the night digging a 6' x 6' x 6' hole under the barracks – which were about two feet off the ground – with an entrenching tool. Needless to say, it was a long night, yet the next day, I was expected to perform everything with the rest of the platoon. I did luck out, as a couple of guys screwed up that day, and had to fill in the hole I had dug.

We were trained on the M-14 and M-16. I had no trouble learning to tear them down and put them together blindfolded. However, I was amazed once we got to the rifle range. There was absolutely no time spent sighting in the weapons, and there was no way of knowing which gun I would have each time. Therefore, when it came time to shoot for a qualifying score, it was ridiculous. I knew I was a very good shot, because I used to shoot pennies out of trees just to impress my girlfriend. Now, I was trying to obtain my marksmanship badge without having any idea where the sights on my gun were set. I did manage to get the sharpshooter badge, but if I could have sighted in and maintained my own gun, I have no doubt I would have earned the expert badge. The funny thing (actually, a sad thing) is that I was never able to sight in any weapon I used in Vietnam. It is a wonder I hit anything.

We occasionally went to town on weekend passes. There was a little town close by named Leesville – but commonly called Fleasville – that was beyond anything I had come to expect. The main businesses in the town were bars and whorehouses. They threw in a junk store here and there, but it was obvious where the

47

bulk of their revenue was generated. On my first and only visit to Leesville, I must admit that I thought it was cool to go into a bar and be served, even though I was well under the legal drinking age. I avoided the whorehouses, would the truth be told, the women looked like they were run hard and put up wet. I returned to the barracks that night, quite drunk, and did not go back to that town again. I figured that I could drink on base, where it was a lot safer.

Basic was the worst experience of my life up to that point. I no longer felt like an individual. It seemed that my thinking was focused entirely upon the well-being of the unit, rather than my own success or failure. I guess that is what the Army really wanted from basic. I was no longer me; I was just part of a machine. I was uneasy about that thought, the thought that I no longer was an individual, composed of my life experience up to that point. This really scared me. I was somehow different now, someone I really did not know or understand. However, I wore the uniform proudly. I received my orders for Fort Lee, Virginia for additional training, and was granted a short leave home.

MOS TRAINING

I was sent home by bus after basic. During my leave, I spent as much time with my fiancé as I could. It was hard for an 18-year-old boy to stay away from his girl so long. The leave soon ended, and I was flown out to Fort Lee, Virginia for Military Occupational Specialty (MOS) training. This is where you are taught the skills needed for performing your specific duties. It was so hard leaving Alice again. I was unsure how long I would be in training, so we really didn't know when we would see each other again.

Fort Lee was like most posts. I learned that this was the center of the Quartermaster Corps in the Army, where everyone was learning to perform some function in the supply train. Getting the supplies out to the troops in the field was the goal of everyone there. I went through two different classes that taught me to order specialized parts. I worked hard and graduated first in both classes. Everything was coming together in my grand plan. Being number one in both classes should pretty much seal my fate in Vietnam; nice air-conditioned offices and a lot of time to have some fun.

ORDERS FOR VIETNAM

Then the orders came, and of course, mine were for Vietnam. Even though I knew that the orders were coming, it still hit me hard. I was going to Vietnam for real. Suddenly, all the images I had seen on TV took on a completely different meaning. I called home to my parents and my fiancée, telling them about the orders. Even though this is what I had planned, it was still a shock, because now it was very real.

I went home on a 30-day leave before shipping out. I was not scared, just very apprehensive. I was with Alice whenever possible. I am not sure how she got any of her homework done. I also said goodbye to a few good friends. My best friend came home on leave after I did, and was getting married before going to Vietnam. He was an airplane mechanic so he was not expecting much action either. Although I had to leave before his wedding, I did not figure the marriage would last even through his twelve-month tour. It has lasted 34 years as I write this.

On our last date, Alice and I went to see John Wayne in *The Green Berets*. It was probably not a good choice, given the fact that I was getting ready to go to 'Nam. I really think that seeing it only worsened her fear about my leaving.

The night before I left, my family, Alice and I went out to the fanciest restaurant in Fort Dodge, about 15 miles from my hometown. You must

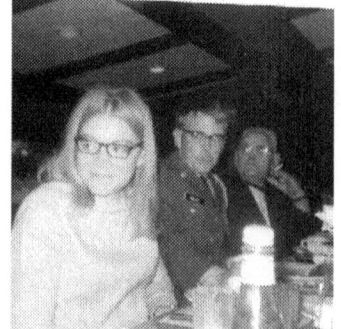

Alice, me and Dad

realize that "fancy" in Iowa means something a lot different than it does in large towns. It is probably the most extravagant restaurant around, but still had a small town "fry it in grease" attitude. My parents, my younger brother and sister, and Alice were there to give me the royal treatment.

The next morning, I left for a Fort in the state of Washington. The name of the place evades me; but I knew that I would be leaving the US for at least a year, a really long time for an 18-year-old. I did not shed a tear or show any fear when I left. Alice's mother had written her teachers a note, saying that she was sick so she could be there to send me off.

It was a very long trip to 'Nam, with stops in Anchorage and Tokyo. We were allowed to get off the plane and stretch our legs, but were surrounded my Military Police. There was no way they were going to let any of us leave a very restricted area and avoid going to Vietnam. It felt like we were prisoners, heading to hell. On both stops we all found the airport bar in short order. Even though most of us were under age, no one ever asked a question.

APRIL 1969

The trip to Alaska and Japan was pretty much a party atmosphere, and we were having a lot of fun. When we left Japan, we all knew the next stop was 'Nam. The planeload of hundreds of soldiers was very quiet. No one ever showed any fear, but we were going to a place that was not totally unknown since we had seen all the pictures on TV and in the print media. But to be actually going there seemed unreal. Until we left Japan, it was as if we were in denial about our destination. Now, we all knew it was for real.

When we landed in Cam Rahn Bay[1], all seemed normal. Then all of a sudden, the field was being mortared. We watched the explosions on the runway, knowing that a direct hit would kill a few hundred GI's all at one time. Needless to say, we all wanted off the plane as it taxied down the runway. We knew we were trapped in this God-forsaken machine and none of us 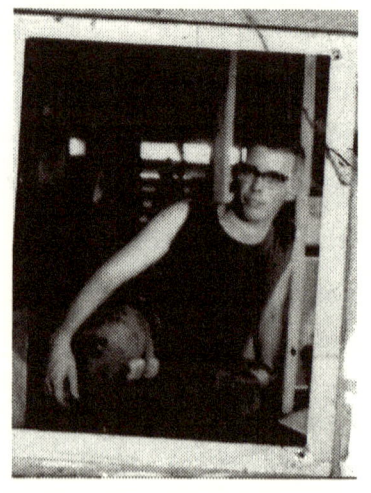 wanted to die before we had even arrived.

The plane taxied to a stop and we all rushed out. The first thing that hit us was the repressive heat. It was like walking into a brick

---

[1] It was not until years later, when reading the letters I had sent my wife while looking for support of my VA claim that I remembered that I had landed in Cam Rahn Bay. I thought that I had landed in Bien Hoa or Tan Son Nhut. I am sure I have landed at all of them but it does show how some facts have been lost over the last thirty years. However, some events – and not necessarily the ones I would choose to remember – have remained as sharp as the day they happened

wall. It took your breath away. After the heat, we were assailed by the stink of Vietnam. It is hard to describe the smell, except to say that it was like rotting vegetation, but much worse. Between the heat and the smell, it was hard to run to cover.

As we were running, we ran past stacks of metal containers. I had seen them on TV – they were caskets going home. I stopped running and walked by them. It was then that I first really felt fear. The mortaring had stopped. Gun ships were lighting up the hills around the airport. I was not afraid of dying at that moment, but I was seeing first-hand that it could happen. I just knew that was the way I would be going home – in an aluminum box. I was afraid. I knew for sure I was now "in country" (a term that simply meant being in Vietnam).

I was shuffled around Cam Rahn Bay and Bien Hoa for what seemed like forever, until I was finally assigned to my unit. We were not told much, but we all knew they were trying to decide which unit to send us to. It was like they were rolling the dice with our lives on the line. That kept the attitudes tense, and the main events of the day were drinking and the occasional fight.

My first exposure to living in a war zone happened to me during the first week or two in one of these bases. The barracks were divided into two man "rooms" by four-foot high plywood. The plywood didn't really afford any privacy but it was much better than an open floor. At least it cut down on the snoring you heard at night. I was assigned to a room with a guy who had been there a few days. Another guy who had flown over with me knew my roommate, and since I did not know anyone, I traded rooms with him so he could spend time with his friend before we were all sent to different units. I ended up in another room at the opposite corner of the barracks from them.

Sometime during the night, an explosion unlike anything I had ever heard in my life awakened me, literally blowing me out of my cot. I was totally disoriented. The air was filled with smoke, dust, and another unfamiliar smell. I could barely hear. I was not sure if I was still alive or not. I crawled out of my room. Instead of turning left, which would have quickly gotten me out of the building, I turned right. I felt the walls as I gradually worked myself down the length of the barracks. Suddenly, the wall was gone. There was enough moon light coming through the large hole in the roof to see that the room was no longer there. I had no clue what was really happening. I just sat there staring out the hole in the roof and into the darkness where the room had been only moments before.

It seemed like a long time, but other soldiers were probably there very quickly with flashlights. That was when I realized that the missing room was the one I had originally been assigned to. I remained sitting. I had no clue what had happened, and even less as to what I should be doing. That doubt was soon removed by an old sergeant. He checked me over, asking if I had been hit by the rocket. The only evidence that I was even close was the blood coming from my ears. He said, "You're okay son. Now help the others down there," and pointed to the missing room.

As I climbed down into the hole, I found it hard to keep a grip on what was left of the walls. As I looked at my hands, I realized that I was slipping on blood. Blood and innards covered everything. Here and there were body parts. The old sergeant threw down a body bag and said, "Throw all the parts into one bag… we'll let graves registration sort them out." There was no way to determine which part belonged to which guy. The rocket had torn the two soldiers apart. I remember getting sick several times as I searched for body parts.

The sun was coming up, giving us a better view of the room. It was more gruesome than I could tell by flashlight. There was just nothing left. The body bag was full of the parts we could find, but the walls were covered in blood and guts. As I took in the image, still very nauseated, I heard my name being called from somewhere above. I yelled back, "Yes sir, I'm Greg Helle." Someone leaned over and said, "What the hell are you doing alive?" I told them the story of swapping the rooms, but I could not tell them the name of the soldier with whom I had traded places. Since everything had been done that could be done, they ordered us all outside for roll call. That is when I noticed that all I had on was my green T-shirt and boxers. My whole body was covered with blood.

After the roll call, I went straight to the showers, took off my T-shirt and boxers, and threw them away. I scrubbed a long time, trying to get the blood off me. Even though the water was frigid, I did not feel it. I only wanted to be clean, but I just could not get clean. I went back to "my" room naked, then got dressed and removed all my belongings. I had no idea what was going to happen, but I just had to get away from those barracks.

I had somehow changed my fate. In my heart, I felt that I was supposed to have died in that room, but that some young man had died in my place. I felt terrible that I was still breathing. The chaplains were around, but I had no time for them. I also know that each of those two men's graves contained parts of each of them. Somehow, this still seems like my fault. This guilt has never left me. I should be dead in my grave, and this other young man should be alive. It was my fault.

Later that day, I was shipped to Long Bien and assigned to my unit. It was a relief to get away from those barracks. Long Bien was a much larger base than I would have believed I would be assigned. It seemed to take forever to get from entrance to Long Bien to my company. The heat and smell were still overpowering.

Several things amazed me as we drove through Long Bien. There was a bridge that seemed to be a hundred feet above the small stream below. This really seemed like overkill, but I found out later that this was sometimes not high enough during the monsoon season. There were many very nice office buildings, but there were also quite a few that had been burned out. Although this post seemed huge, it did not look or feel safe. I knew I was not in a firebase, where combat was a part of everyday life, but the fear was still there.

MAY 1969

For the first couple of weeks, I really did not perform any task close to what I had been trained for. As a "newbie," I was treated to all the fun jobs. Newbies were generally not trusted; since they usually did not have command of the weapons we used and had not been tested in a battle situation. We were also affectionately called "FNG's (Fucking New Guy.) The prevailing attitude was that newbies were little more than "meat," and would probably get themselves – not to mention some of their fellow squad members – killed. It took a while to gain the trust of the others, so the newbies stuck together a lot of the time. It was great once I had been in country long enough to start hassling the newbies who were arriving.

The worst job was burning the human waste from the latrines, which were little more than platforms atop half of a fifty-gallon drum. We had to pull these drums out from under the platforms and use fuel oil to burn the waste. Besides having to stir it (the smell is very difficult to describe), we were enveloped in a dark cloud of

smoke. Just pulling out the drums filled with urine and feces was bad enough, but usually there was enough of a drop so that you could not help being splashed in the process. Like everybody else, I hated this job with a passion. The only relief was that some of the buildings had real plumbing that

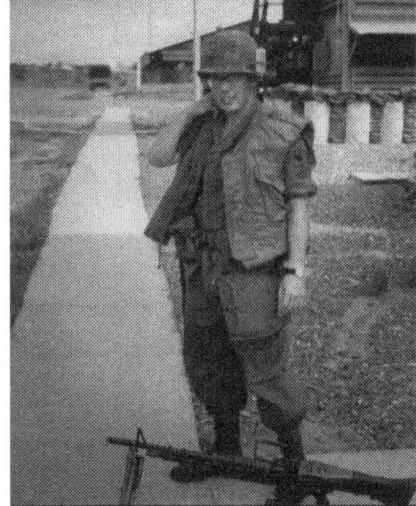

probably cut down on the amount we had to burn. I recall thinking that it was too bad that they did not put plumbing in the barracks.

Another never-ending task was keeping the company area cleaned. This was handled just the way it was on stateside bases. We had to rake the dust so it had nice clean rows, and even in Vietnam, they liked to have their rocks painted white. Everyone got the job of doing this at one time or another. It seemed like a ridiculous thing to be doing in a war zone, but I never did figure out why the Army did a lot of things.

We also spent a significant amount of time on the wire, which is what we "affectionately" called the perimeter of the base. Most areas had bunkers built into berms, with concertina wire strung out in front of the bunkers and berms. This concertina wire was our first line of defense. I wasn't happy the first time they took us out to the perimeter. After all, we were all trained as clerks, not as combat soldiers. We were classified as non-combatants — what a joke. The first time out, we were given our only training on weapons that we had not seen before, much less qualified with. In basic, we were trained on the M-14, M-16, and grenades, and given some basic hand-to-hand combat instruction. All of a sudden, I was carrying an M-60 machine gun, and some had M-79 grenade launchers. Then they pointed out the claymore mines. These little gems had folding steel legs that stuck into the ground, holding the mine vertically, with the curved side facing towards the enemy. A long wire connected a blasting cap stuck into the mine to a hand detonator. During an attack, you were supposed to squeeze the firing handle, setting off the mine, sending hundreds of small steel balls hurtling toward the enemy, with devastating effects.

I really knew then that I was in a different world. We had a few hours that afternoon when they gave us training on these weapons. We shot the M-60 machine gun, learned how to change the barrel when it got hot enough to make the weapon malfunction, got to shoot the M-79 grenade launcher at an old APC (armored personnel carrier), and were given basic instruction of the use of the claymores. They also briefly taught us about some of the tricks that the "gooks" would use to get through the wire. We learned what satchel charges were, and were told to make sure the claymores were facing the right direction. By that evening, we were "experts" on the use of these weapons, or at least we were told that we better have learned quickly because they might save our lives tonight. This all happened in the space of about four hours in the sweltering afternoon heat. This training was, to say the least, not very reassuring

Behind our bunker area were what seemed like several hundred small bunkers. We were informed that our assigned area was just outside the ammunition dump, a favorite place for the "gooks" to attack. Everything just kept getting better.

We were given the password for the night and assigned a bunker. There were three of us newbies there and an "experienced" E5 from our company. The heat index of the bunker must have been well over 100 degrees, and it smelled like urine. There were two cots in the back, or at least two places where we could lie down on a wood platform for sleep that usually was not possible. Entering the bunker was like going through a tunnel. It was very much like being trapped.

We were served a "fantastic" meal of C-rations. It was food only in the sense that it had some calories and perhaps enough nutrition to keep you alive. Beyond that, there was no redeeming value in the rations. Throughout my tour, I never changed my mind about C-rations. I hated them.

As night fell, it was soon apparent that we could not see anything in front of us. The night scope soon became our best friend. At least with that scope, we had a chance to see someone coming. We had a four-man bunker, so there were always two on duty. If you were off duty, you got to lie down on one of the plywood cots and attempt to get some sleep, which required that you had complete confidence in those on duty. It was a long time before I was able to sleep on the wire. I would lie down and close my eyes, but every one of my senses seemed on alert. It did not take much of a sound for me to be up and ready. At least the first night was quiet.

Much of the other early duty was very mundane. The only thing we lacked was sleep. Often we would be in charge of checking the papers of the civilians entering the post. There were many civilians who did a wide range of duties around the post. The civilians were the main ones building the post's defenses. It always amazed me that we let Vietnamese build our defenses, since I could not tell a South Vietnamese from a Viet Cong or North Vietnamese, and seriously doubted that any of my fellow soldiers could, either. So we sat on the line, knowing that in all probability, they had us zeroed in with their mortars. In addition, there was always that fact that gnawed on you — they knew where *we* were, but we had no clue where *they* were. Anyway, we tried to act official and at least make sure they weren't bringing in a satchel charge, and had papers that looked somewhat official.

I have no clue how many nights I spent on the wire that month, but I did not see my cot that often. There were nights when a few shots were fired both ways, but not a lot of action most nights. There was, however, one night when we were being hit pretty hard. In my memory, firefights seemed as if they lasted for hours when in reality, they usually only lasted 15-20 minutes. As we were fighting out the front of the bunker, I caught sight of a "gook" out of the corner of my eye. He was coming under the wire. I took aim and watched him for what seemed like a long time. I knew he probably would have a satchel charge that would kill all of us, so I could not think of him in human terms. My duty was clear. I put my weapon on full automatic and emptied my clip into him. There was no life left. The firefight was over pretty quickly, but I had to watch that body for the rest of the night. In the morning, I had to help remove the body and body parts from the wire. I was physically and mentally sick. I knew my Ten Commandments well. Now, I had killed, and I could not call back my bullets. I felt somehow evil inside. Even though my duty as a soldier was to kill the enemy, I was struggling inside. Even as my fellow soldiers congratulated me, I felt no hatred for this person. There was only compassion. In my heart, there was no way around it; I had sinned.

I was finally assigned my permanent duty, as aide to a full colonel, taking him anywhere he wanted, going wherever he went, and solving problems for him. Several of my classmates were doing the jobs we were trained for, but I was going to be doing something very different. It somehow seemed odd that, having graduated number one in both my specialized training classes, I would be assigned different duties more logically given to one of the other guys who had graduated under me. I just figured this was another Army SNAFU ("situation normal, all fucked up"). One of my counselors brought up the idea that my record indicated that I was more intelligent than some of the others, and that is what the colonel wanted. I will never know, and had nothing to say about it. The Army was big on following orders, not understanding or questioning them.

JUNE 1969

The colonel and I got along very well. He had come up through the enlisted ranks, so he was a little less Army than most career officers were. That really gave me a lot of flexibility in the job and allowed me to see much of Vietnam. I was able to travel often with the colonel. We made frequent trips to Saigon. The colonel knew I loved photography, so sometimes he would drive so I could get pictures. It was so funny when soldiers realized a full colonel was driving an E-4 or E-5 around. They probably wondered which of us they were supposed to salute.

One of the things I noticed soon after arrival in country was that the EM (enlisted men's) club was very close to the company area. I had been there on several occasions, but now it became a daily part of my life. For one thing, this was one of the only places you could get your beer cold. I started by occasionally having a few beers with friends, but after I had been there a very short time, it became a passion. I started drinking as often as possible, and usually as much as possible. My friends introduced me to marijuana, and sometimes we were able to get hold of marijuana laced with opium. After only a month and a half in Vietnam, I was already so filled with guilt that I wanted to dull the emotions any way I could. If I was not officially on duty, you would usually find me drunk, high, or both. I had broken – and was continuing to break – the laws of my God, and this was my escape.

I was learning very quickly that emotions were unwanted. We were told that if the US government had wanted us to have feelings, it would have issued them to us with our uniforms. Like most soldiers, I used alcohol and drugs to numb the emotions that I did not want to feel for what I had seen and what I had done. We spent our time "comfortably numb," as the song said, never talked about anything. When one of ours was wounded or killed, we just shrugged it off. "Shit happens."

One June night in 1969, I had been out drinking with my buds. I do not remember if it was in the EM club or just sitting behind a bunker. Wherever it was, I went to my bunk intoxicated. My room was on the second floor, southwest corner. Some time during the night, I was awakened. I realized that my boxers were being pulled off, but beyond that I had no clue what was happening. Then I remember my legs being forced apart. I remember trying to turn over, but being forced back down. I will always remember his face. Then I felt him forcing himself into me. I remember the pain. I can remember his entering me repeatedly, but not being able to do anything about it. It seemed like he pounded me forever.

The next thing I remember, it was morning. I was naked, and what had happened the night before came clearly to my mind. This event, and my attacker's name and face, I would never forget. He was a fellow soldier who bunked across the hall from me. I remember hating him. I remember giving him hate looks that I know he understood. I wanted to kill him; I have no idea why I didn't. I had my chances. I often wish I had.

Yet the thought of reporting this attack did not even enter my mind. I knew I had been unable to stop what had happened to me; I just lay there and took it. I knew I was drunk and that prevented me from fucking this guy over. But somehow I felt that I was to blame for letting this happen to me. I was confused and ashamed.

I was also well aware that I was in the "man's" Army. I felt that my own personal weakness had caused this to happen, and being weak was not an option. I could not face my buds if they were to find out. I have no idea if they could have medically proved it had even happened, and if that were the case it would be my word against his.

Another problem was that my attacker was Hispanic, and the Hispanic soldiers stuck close together. Of course we all carried guns. We all knew about eliminating bad officers; friendly fire was not always friendly. I was well aware that an "accident" could happen to me at any time. I knew that if I reported him, I would be a marked man.

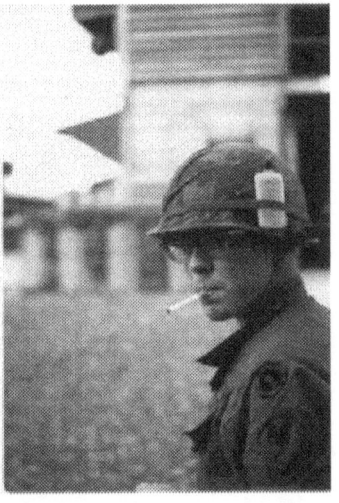

After this, my world totally changed forever. I knew before I got to 'Nam I could not trust the VC (Viet Cong). I learned soon after arriving that you could not trust *any* Vietnamese, man, woman, or child; in Saigon, I soon found it easy to point my .45 (weapon) at women and children – fully prepared to pull the trigger if they came close to my jeep. And now I could not even trust my fellow soldiers. I did not know who would hurt me. I was totally alone. I made sure to cover my own back, as I could not trust anyone else to keep me alive. I didn't allow anyone holding a loaded gun behind me. I feared my own comrades more than I feared the enemy. I kept a knife strapped to my bunk at all times. I was not going to be attacked again. I still have a knife close to my bed; even after all these years, my own bedroom is not safe. Nowhere is safe, and I am always afraid.

Thirty years later, I located a friend who served with me. Even after all those years, he remembers the change in my personality around that time. The first week in July 1969, I wrote my fiancée that I would not be going into the ministry. I felt that I had very little to live for, and that there was no redemption for me.

But I still needed to fight my war.

JULY 1969

As I mentioned earlier, one of the "perks" of working for my colonel was that I got to travel all over Vietnam. When we were in Long Bien, I actually got to work in an air-conditioned office. However, the colonel was always concerned that supplies got to the troops in the front lines, so we very frequently flew in and out of firebases. Of course, the colonel always got the best hooch (quarters) and food, while I usually ended up eating C-rations and sleeping in a bunker or hole in the ground.

Most of the firebases were manned by grunts, who referred to me as a REMF (rear echelon mother fucker). Since I was not a grunt, they usually had fun with me. The worst was when they assigned me the listening post. I would go out about 100 yards in front of the perimeter. My job was to be out there to give early warning of an attack. I had my M-16, .45, bayonet, and one flare. My task was to listen for any enemy activity. I would have to engage (exchange fire with) any that got too close

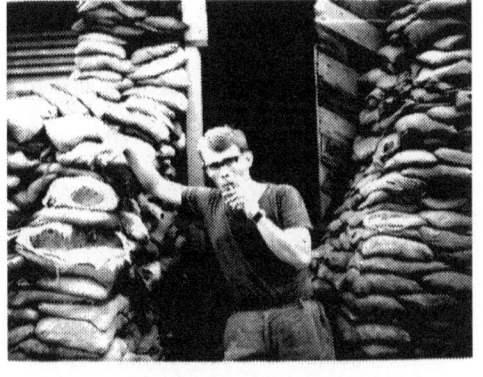

Me at the rear of a bunker

to me. The flare was shot to tell the guys back at the firebase that I was coming back in, after which I had to make a dead run back inside the perimeter, hoping that I could get there before either side shot me.

Somewhere in Vietnam, in some lonely firebase(s), two more events occurred in July 1969 that continues to change my life. I have no idea of the chronology of these events, but through years of therapy, I do know they both happened in July.

One night I was lucky enough to be in a firebase with bunkers. Somehow, having all those sandbags around me made me feel safer. I was usually on second watch because I could go to sleep earlier than most people did, and tonight was no exception. It was the middle of the night and I was on duty with another young soldier; he couldn't have been more than 18 or 19. We were discussing the normal things – all the girls we'd had at home, and all the whores we'd had in country. It was simple talk, but helped us pass the long night. It was a quiet and boring night; nothing was happening up or down the line. We were looking out the firing slit in the front of the bunker when I heard one shot. My buddy fell back against the wall of the bunker. I turned around and he fell into my arms as I sunk down into a corner of the bunker. I was not sure what had happened. He looked like he was sleeping. There was a small mark on his forehead, but as I turned his head around, there was nothing left of the back of his head. I felt his blood and brains as they soaked my uniform. I could not let go of him, and I held him close for what seemed like hours. I did not want to admit that he was gone. I did not want him to be dead. We were shoulder to shoulder, and there was no reason he was shot instead of me. The other two in the bunker took over control of the bunker. I had tears running down my face as I held him. I should have died. It should have been me.

The sergeant of the guard soon came into the bunker. He pulled my buddy away from me and laid him in a corner. I was still sitting terrified in the corner. The sergeant shoved my M-16 back in my hands and told me to "get back into the fucking war." He made me empty my clip into the nothingness in front of us. I remained on duty the rest of the night with my buddy lying behind me. I kept looking back at him. In the morning, they came in, put him in a body bag, threw him on a truck, and it was all over. Did I know his name? I am not sure. We had probably just met that night, but the guilt will be with me always. There was no reason for him to die and not me.

Another night in some firebase somewhere in Vietnam, I was pulling duty on the wire again. Most nights were boring, but that night, all hell broke loose. The gooks were hitting hard up and down the line. Somewhere on the line, they broke through the perimeter. The bunker was built to fight forward; the entrance was basically a tunnel at the rear. Since there were gooks behind the line, I went out the back to ensure that we would not be blown. I walked through the tunnel, and, as I turned, I came face to face with a VC. We were only a couple of feet apart. I think we were both shocked, but I was lucky and pulled my trigger first. My M-16 was on full auto and I emptied the clip, watching the shock in his eyes as my bullets tore his body apart. We were so close that his blood spattered my uniform. I was still shaking. I knew he was dead, but I was so afraid. I locked and loaded and spent the rest of the night protecting the rear of my bunker. The fighting did not last long. The gook I killed looked like he was not more than sixteen. I was so grateful when the sun came up and this was finally over. His body was removed, and life went back to "normal." – except it was never again to be normal. I had killed a second time.

AUGUST-OCTOBER 1969

I know in my heart that I had killed others. In most firefights, there were so many people firing that we never knew who actually killed the gooks. Most times, we could not even find bodies the next day. We would find blood and some body parts, but not bodies. That, in and of itself, was more unsettling than I could ever have imagined.

It was at this point that I totally shut down emotionally. I was not going to let anything hurt me anymore. I did not want friends, because friends die. I did not want to feel any compassion for the enemy or for anyone. I just wanted to be left alone and wanted to be responsible for only myself. My alcohol and drug use increased, and I was even using on duty. Several of us would "requisition" beer from the depot and keep it immediately available in our rooms. Warm or even hot beer was acceptable. After a half dozen, the temperature did not even matter, anyway. All that mattered was suppressing any emotions.

The months of August through October of 1969 are a mystery to me. I have no clue where I was or what I did during those months. There is no way for me to know at this time if it was just so boring that there was nothing to remember, or that I have blocked out other incidents.

Although many of the memories of Vietnam are now nightmares, it was not all bad. I do remember the Philippine rock groups who would come to our company area and entertain those of us who were lucky enough to have the night off duty. They sang all the good songs of the time, albeit with a heavy accent. We did not care. We were generally drunk enough to sing over them, anyway. The girls they had with them were the big attractions. I have tons of pictures of those girls, mostly taken while I was lying on the stage trying to get the good shots.

Every vice imaginable was easily available in 'Nam. There were whores everywhere. It was also easy to obtain drugs of any kind. I never did go beyond smoking marijuana and some opium, but many soldiers were hooked on stronger drugs like heroin. The military went through the motions of trying to control the drugs but never made any serious effort to stop the flow of drugs or to help those soldiers who had become addicted. The military did not even try to keep track of the morphine that was used. Much of it was used to get high. It was not often that I did not have morphine on me. This was all part of the way soldiers like myself buried the emotions of the war. Most of the time, I also had marijuana and naturally, if I could figure out a way, I had some beer with me as well.

I remember one event that is funny now, but it was pretty serious when it happened. We loved stealing jeeps and taking them for joy rides. The higher the rank of the officer, the more fun we had with his jeep. We would just have fun and then dump it somewhere. One time, we rolled the jeep. We all got out pretty much unharmed, but after that jeep rolled down that big hill, it was totaled, and we all knew that if we owned up to the deed, we would be forced to pay for the jeep. That was not an option on the amount of pay we were getting, so we decided upon a different course. We blew up the jeep and watched it burn. It was now just another casualty of war. We hitched a ride back to our company area and played dumb when the poop hit the fan.

NOVEMBER 1969

While the majority of November is a blur like the previous months, there was one night – November 28, 1969 – that will haunt me forever. We were on the wire as usual in a four-man bunker. One of the men was a newbie, and I do not think he had seen much – if any – action. The night started as usual. We checked all the weapons, and then settled down for a boring night. Sometime that night, all hell broke loose. We were being mortared and we knew from the night scopes that there were plenty of gooks moving our way. So we threw everything we had at them. The firing slit was not large enough for four, so I went out to the berm with my M-16 and fought from there. They were coming at us fast. I think that was the only time that I actually had to use the claymores. Thankfully, air support was called in. The gun ship we called the Jolly Green Giant[2] came through the area with its miniguns, which were modern (and devastating) versions of the old Gattling gun. The sky was filled with tracer rounds, and the bullets landed so close to each other that nothing could survive. That saved our butts that night. We were very close to being overrun, and without the air support, I think they would have broken through the line and maybe gotten as far as blowing up part of the ammo dump.

I came back into the bunker. The adrenaline high was fantastic. We had held and no one in the bunker had been hurt. The barrel of the M-60 was shot, but we did not care. We were alive and well.

---

[2] A heavily armed air force C-47 aircraft used in supporting ground troops.

That is all that mattered. It was a party atmosphere in the bunker with high-fives everywhere.

The newbie told us he was going outside for a piss. This was not unusual and much preferred to pissing in a corner of the bunker. Most bunkers smelled very strongly of urine. There often were times that it was impossible to leave the post, so there was no option but to urinate on the floor. No one noticed that he went out with the M-79 in his hands.

Suddenly, we heard the distinctive *thunk* of the M-79. I ran out of the bunker to find that this newbie had shot himself in the head with the grenade launcher. Most of his head was blown away, but the live shell was still embedded in what was left of it. Because of the danger involved with removing the live shell, I was on guard duty the rest of the night waiting for ordnance to come and take care of that live grenade. That gave me a lot of time to think about what had happened. He must have been so scared during the firefight. Hell, we all were. Why didn't I notice that he was not celebrating like the rest of us? Why didn't I see him leave with the '79? I was the ranking Non-Commissioned Officer in the bunker, so I was responsible for him. It was my fault. I should have stopped him. I had fucked up, and now he was dead. Years later, with the help of a man I served with, I was able to search through databases and find the name of this young man. He was only 21 at the time. In July 2003, I was finally able to get a rubbing of his name on the Vietnam Memorial Wall. In respect to him and his family, I am not going to disclose his identity. I still feel somehow responsible for his death. His name should not be on that Wall.

In the morning, ordnance made it out and removed the live shell. Then we just bagged him and threw him on a truck. That was the end of the story. We went back to our company area one short, and no one said a word. I have no clue what the other two men were thinking. It was just one of those "tough shit" or sin loi" (Vietnamese for "too bad") times that were never discussed. Even though we had been up all night, we needed booze and drugs to get any kind of sleep.

My friend was the company clerk, and had to write the lies back to the parents of this young man. There was no way that the company commander was going to tell them that their son had committed suicide. He was just another casualty of the war, sent home and forgotten.

DECEMBER 1969

There are some memories that have stayed with me that happened in December. I remember when Bob Hope and his troupe came through Long Bien in 1969. He and the others helped soften the negative feelings we had about being so far from home at Christmas time. I will miss him and all that he has done for soldiers through the decades.

Christmas 1969 also brought another surprise for us. The Jewish soldiers in our company volunteered to take line duty on Christmas Eve. They were willing to put their lives on the line so that the Christians could celebrate Christmas. My heart still beats faster when I think of the potential sacrifice of these brothers. We made sure to volunteer during one of their holidays. It was the least we could do. Of course, we celebrated Christmas like everything else — with heavy doses of booze and drugs. I knew of very few who actually went to the services in the chapel.

Another fond memory of that Christmas was of the cookies sent to me by Alice and her best friend. One of my favorites was a Norwegian cookie called a sun bakel, which was basically a sugar cookie pressed into a tin. The ones that did not break were carefully packed for me, and the girls ate the failures. By the time the box of "perfect" cookies arrived, there was nothing left except crumbles. It did not matter; everyone loved eating them with a spoon. It still hits me that something as simple as a tin of crumbled up cookies could make Christmas so special.

JANUARY 1970

There are some new memories coming out in therapy about January 1970. Starting in October 2002, I was starting to have more – and new – nightmares. I thought at first that the anniversary of the newbies death, which was coming in November, was the problem. However, the feelings, and the new dream, continued. In this dream, I saw myself grabbing someone from behind around his forehead. I then could feel myself cutting his throat. I could feel the muscles being cut, and the warmth of his blood. The dream seems to always end with me dropping his limp body.

I can't help but wonder whether the horrible dream could be a memory of something that had actually happened. Could I have been put in a position of having to do this? The war was filled with so many events that are unthinkable to any civilized person, so there is a possibility. Did it really happen? My psychologist is convinced that it is not a false memory. At this point, I am not convinced, but it does explain some things that happened much later in my life. There is something that is more disturbing about killing someone with my hands instead of a weapon. Every time I have this nightmare, it is very real and continues to haunt me for a long time. Having killed someone with my own hands, feeling his life seep out of him, is a reality that I am not sure I can handle. I dread the reemergence of the memories of this incident coming back into my life. There is just something about taking a life by my own hands that is much worse than anything that has come to light before.

And now, I wonder if there are any other horrors still hidden in my subconscious, waiting to invade my dreams – and my hope of peace.

FEBRUARY-MAY 1970

This is another period of lost memories. Sometime during this period, I had five days of R&R (rest & recuperation) in Bangkok, Thailand. I know I was there because I have several hundred pictures I took of different places I visited. I just do not remember much about being there. I do remember that when we landed, the Army made us go through an orientation before they would let us loose. They were handing out quart bottles of Thai beer. I do not remember the orientation or getting to my hotel. Maybe that was the purpose of the beer. I have no idea what its alcohol percentage was, but it kicked ass compared to the 3.2 stuff they gave us in 'Nam.

The only other things I remember about Bangkok are that there were street vendors everywhere. Most of them were selling food, but a lot were selling junk to the GI's. Actually, most of the food I tried was good. I did not have a clue how safe it was, or even what was in it, but anything was an improvement over Army cooking and C-rations. While I was there, I had a personal driver. He would take us anywhere we wanted at any time of the day or night. As I remember, it cost me $15 for the week. I remember too that prostitution was legal in Bangkok. We would go to these parlors where there was a glassed-in room, and would sit around the edge of the room drinking their free booze. All we had to do was pick out one of the women we liked. It was a different world, as intense in its pleasures as the war was in its ugliness. All too soon, however, I was back in 'Nam.

Sometime during this period, we had a company commander who was an airborne ranger lieutenant. I have no clue why they would assign him to what was basically a supply company. He tried to pull all the airborne ranger crap on us, with very little success. One night when I was on the line, he showed up. Authorized personnel on the line knew the password for the night, and our orders were to treat anyone else like the enemy. The lieutenant tried to enter my bunker, and I stopped him and asked for the password. He was giving me shit about being court martialed if I did not let him pass. He did not know the answer, so I locked and loaded my M-16 and ordered him to get down on the ground spread-eagled. I think he knew I was serious. The guys in the bunker called into the line commander and let him know that we were holding an unauthorized person. When the commander came, it was great. The lieutenant was still threatening to court martial me for the way I handled him. The commander let him know in no uncertain terms that if *anyone* was going to get court martialed, it would be him, and that a report of the incident would be sent to his superior. I never heard a word from him about it, and he never showed up on the line again.

This same lieutenant later traded one of our night vision scopes for a fifty caliber machine gun, which he had mounted on his jeep. We really depended upon our night scopes on the line, so it really pissed off the company that he had done this. Besides, if he had shot that .50 cal, he probably would have rolled the jeep. Then, rather than get in trouble for having an unauthorized weapon discovered on his jeep during an upcoming inspection, he removed the .50 cal and buried it. This was the last straw for us. Rumor has it that *somebody* wanted to take out this asshole, and booby-trapped his hooch with fragmentary grenades. I am not sure how it happened, but apparently the trap was foiled. However, the lieutenant was shipped out the next day to places unknown. I wish I remembered his name, so I could see if he actually survived Vietnam.

Sometime during this period, I extended my tour. Each extension was six months. At the time, I had no clue why I did this (a common mystery among guys who re-up). I could have been home in April, but instead I chose to stay.

JUNE-JULY 1970

June and July were magical months for me. I had asked for a 45-day leave, but the Army would only give me 30 days. I complained but it had no effect. Even so, after being in Vietnam for 14 months, I was finally going home. Not just going home; I was going to be married to my high school sweetheart. I do not remember much about the trip home, but I am fairly sure that I did go through Oakland, California.

I remember being at the airport waiting to fly home. I was in my Class A uniform, and despite all that had happened over the last fourteen months, I was proud to be coming home. I guess I expected to come home a hero. However, the reaction I experienced in the San Francisco airport was totally the opposite. The airport seemed to be full of protesters. They had no clue what my job was, they just knew I was a soldier returning from Vietnam. I was spat upon and called all sorts of names, including baby killer. This was not the country I had left. This did not seem to be my country at all any more. However, soon I was back with my family and the love of my life.

I didn't think about it at the time, but now that I look back, this was a year after my rape. I still had told no one, of course.

My family and sweetheart knew that I had been trained as a supply clerk when I went to 'Nam. During my whole tour in 'Nam, I always wrote home that I was a clerk sitting in an air-conditioned office. That was not a total lie, because I did do some of that kind of work. I just did not tell them the whole truth.

I remember my dad and mom being so happy that I came home alive and unhurt. I was home ten days before the wedding. I had a tough time telling them (and my sweetheart) that I would be returning to 'Nam. In an attempt to soften the news about my having to go back, I told them I had a 45-day leave, rather than the mere 30 days I had been granted. Needless to say, my folks were not happy anyway. At that time, a girl could sign a marriage certificate at 19, but a male needed to be 21 to get married without a parent's signature. I remember my dad refusing to sign the certificate because I was going back. He told me that he got me back alive this time, but there were no promises I would come back alive if I went back. I had to sweet-talk my mom into signing. After all, the wedding was all planned. Alice had planned everything while I was in 'Nam. She would get upset when she would write me and ask my opinion about something concerning the wedding. A month or so later she would get my reply, which was that I did not care. Actually there was some concern whether we would even like each other after being so far apart for fourteen months. As it turned out, that was not a problem then, and thankfully never has been.

Although I did not realize it at the time, I was very sexually aggressive with Alice from the time I came home. She really wanted to wait till the honeymoon, but there was no way I was going to let that happen. Now I know it had to do with what happened a year earlier. I wanted her to know for certain that I was heterosexual, even though she had no clue what had happened to me, and wasn't harboring any doubts. I really did not have any idea of the effect that incident had on me until many years later.

We had a wonderful wedding. However, the temperature in the church was close to that of Vietnam. The guys' tuxedos were drenched by the end of the ceremony, but we were happy. I did not want to leave the reception, as there were people there I had not seen in over a year. But we were made to leave. I did not have a car, so my father-in-law, Loren, allowed us to use his brand new car. The car was full of

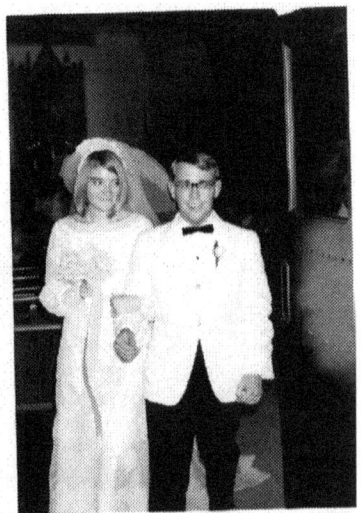

balloons. As we popped the balloons, we soon discovered that they were full of rice. Even our luggage ended up being so full of rice that we kept finding traces of it years later. We had a one-week honeymoon at a small unimpressive cottage on Spirit Lake, where we had first met. Alice's dad was upset we did not use *their* cabin at Spirit Lake, but it did not have a shower, and I wanted everything to be as nice as possible for Alice.

I did take a 45-day leave, and we spent most of that time visiting friends and family and having a lot of sex. It was a great time, but went by way too quickly, and before I knew it, I was again leaving for Vietnam. It was harder leaving a wife than it was a girlfriend. In so many ways, I did not want to return to 'Nam, but I knew I had no choice.

RETURNING TO VIETNAM

I was apprehensive, since I knew I had been AWOL (absent without leave) for 15 days. I reported to Oakland, and nothing much was said. The flight back went through Hawaii and Guam. We spent several days in Guam due to airplane problems. They put us in a hotel right across from a whorehouse. I drank a lot there, but I never again would be with a prostitute. We finally landed in Bien Hoa, and I was transported back to my company. The company commander wanted to bring me up on court martial charges, but my colonel told him that I had gone home, gotten married, and actually came back so he ought to leave me alone. They just added the 15 days to my tour.

For some reason, I took my college entrance exam in 'Nam. I think the main reason I took the exam was that Alice was going to college. The day of my exam, I had been out on the line for three sleepless days. I went to the testing station, laid my M-16 on the table, and took the test. (I am sure the test proctor was a little nervous with all the weapons in the room.) As I was so sleep-deprived, I knew my score sucked.

It was not long after I had gotten back to 'Nam that I found out Alice was pregnant with my child. Now, I had a wife, and would soon be a dad. You might have thought I would have been eager to get home. Instead, it felt as if I had nothing else to expect from life – so I extended for another six months. I did not know it at the time, but I was preparing for death. I wanted a soldier's death.

During this tour, I would volunteer for anything. On the wire, I would sit on top of the bunkers and smoke marijuana, expecting that a sniper would take me out. I wanted to die. However, the gooks would not kill me. Shells hit all around me, but would not hit home. The damn "gooks" had to be the worst shots ever. I saw other people die, but never me. I was getting so frustrated, I extended for another six months. I wanted the gooks to have as much opportunity to kill me as possible.

I never told Alice that I volunteered to stay in 'Nam longer. She would have killed me, and I think my dad would have helped. But I did not want to come home alive. I was stuffing[3] so much pain already; I did not want to have to survive. The things I would do on the line included removing the stuffing from my flack jacket and filling it with beer. I always carried morphine with me, and often the first thing I would do after the OD (officer of the day) left was to inject myself. I spent very little time inside the bunker. Instead I would sit on top of the bunker or berm drinking and smoking marijuana. I am sure this scared the newbies, but I was no longer concerned about the people I was in charge of for the defense of the perimeter. I knew that no one would tell the brass what I was doing, because I was always a good fighter if we were hit. I do not remember anyone getting hurt because of my attitude.

I totally ignored mortar or rocket attacks. We would often be mortared on the line, and I would just watch the explosions. None

---

[3] "Stuffing" was a term I learned in treatment. This meant stuffing feelings and emotions so deep down in our subconscious that they were prevented from becoming part of our daily functioning. This was very important to keep functioning and helped us stay alive in 'Nam. All that we saw and did was not allowed to surface in our conscious memory. Many of us were able to keep these feelings, emotions, and memories stuffed for decades.

of them hit close enough to get me. When I was in the barracks on the main base, I would just go out to the balcony and watch the rocket and mortar hits. Again, they were never close enough to hurt or kill me.

Another thing that was useless to me was the chaplain on base. It would seem natural to go to the chaplain for advice and forgiveness, but it soon became obvious that the chaplains were just like any other officer. Our chaplain wanted to be addressed by his rank. Like all of the chaplains he was true military, and just told me to keep doing my job. So much for being comforted about the realities of the war. I never had communion during the war; it simply was not important to me any more.

In December 1970, they were downsizing the troops in country and I was offered the opportunity to go home. By this time, Alice had suffered a miscarriage. I missed her, and it was obvious that my fate was not to die here. So I accepted their offer. I sent Alice a telegram telling her the news, but she did not get it. When I called from San Francisco on December 23, therefore, it was a real shock to her. This time, after I processed out of Oakland, I immediately purchased some cheap civilian clothes. Only after changing into the civilian clothes did I go to the San Francisco airport. I did my best to blend into the crowd. I landed in Minneapolis on Christmas Eve, but my wife was looking for a soldier and missed me at first. Alice's brother Fred was with her, and though he was only 16 at the time, he drove us home to Iowa in a snowstorm, and I made it there for the traditional Christmas dinner. My mother-in-law, Lucille, would not let anyone eat until we got home. As I finished the meal,

I noticed that there was still Vietnam dirt under my fingernails. I was not home yet, at least in my heart.

TERMINAL DUTY

I spent the last eight months of my enlistment back at Fort Lee, Virginia. It was very boring. Alice dropped out of school for the semester, so I did not have to live on the post. The amazing thing about being there was that so many of the enlisted men and officers were scared of those who had been in 'Nam. We were very disrespectful to the officers, and nothing ever happened. They knew that most of us just wanted to get out of the Army.

The Vietnam vets stayed together spending many of our nights drinking, smoking pot, and just being on the edge. I was assigned to a company, but they only gave me company duty once in the eight months I was there.

I was accepted – on probationary status – by Iowa State University, the school my wife had been attending. Soon I was out of the Army, three months early, to attend college. I was not sure I wanted college, but I was damn sure that I wanted out of the Army.

CHAPTER FIVE

COMING HOME

While in country, it seemed that every soldier's dream from day one was to come home. Everyone carried pictures of girlfriends or wives. Even pictures of Mom and Dad, as well as the siblings, got passed around so we all could brag. We were from all areas of the country and a variety of backgrounds. We would talk endlessly about our homes and the people in our lives. Of course, since most of us were under twenty, we felt compelled to brag about our successes with multiple girls back home. We all knew that most of it was bragging, but it made for some good conversations.

We all had our own little mementos from home to remind us that we were going to make it back. Besides the photos, there was always something else. Mine was the Iowa Flag. It had flown over the statehouse in Des Moines, and was sent to me by the governor. This gave me an identity, and was like a piece of home that I could carry with me. Thirty years after the war, I was able to get a picture of the governor and me with the flag. The flag is still precious, but so now is the picture of me with the governor who sent that flag to me in 'Nam.

Music also became a significant part of our culture, even though most of us could not sing. Some of the songs were from home, but the current pop music was also a big part of our lives. The military would not play certain songs, but they were smuggled from home. I think the favorite was a song by the Animals that has a part that says, "We've got to get out of this place, if it's the last thing we ever do."

We all knew that the military radio would not play songs that they considered detrimental to the war effort, or that they thought might be demoralizing to the soldiers. This did not make much sense, since we could always listen to the propaganda from Hanoi. The newspaper "Stars and Stripes" was also just a propaganda paper. Some of us would get papers from home, or letters that told us what really was happening at home. We knew that many members of our own generation were protesting the war. We knew we were being called baby killers, and that some students were killed as they protested. The world we called home was rapidly changing, and all we were doing was trying to stay alive. We followed orders to do things that were not what we would normally even consider doing, but we were in a war, supposedly defending democracy. We were too young to understand politics. We were just soldiers.

As I mentioned in the previous chapter, my perspective on coming home changed drastically when I came home on leave in 1970. On my journey home, I was feeling proud in my uniform, adorned with the medals I had been awarded. I had heard about the protestors harassing soldiers and spitting on them, but I was not willing at that point to accept that version of reality. I expected, in my own naive way, that I would get a hero's welcome. However, upon arriving at the airport, I felt like I was the enemy. The protestors called me all sorts of names. They spat on me. Some people are now saying this never happened; believe me, it did. I did not feel like a soldier coming home from doing his duty to his country. I felt like a murderer. I had done something that made me into a pariah in my own country.

When I was home on leave in 1970, it was as if no one really cared where I had been. There were no "Thank you's" or other recognition that I had been to war for fourteen months. I just stuck close to my family and my fiancée. There was some safety with family that I did not feel with the general public. I do not know what I really expected, but after what I had gone through, I suppose I expected some kind of recognition from my hometown. Instead, I was shunned, and I felt that I was no longer welcome in the "civilized" world. I knew at that point that I could not go home again, because the world I knew had disappeared in my absence.

When I came home for the last time, I actually had to sneak home. I did not want anyone to know that I was a soldier, much less a Vietnam vet. I could no longer be proud of my service. I had to make sure no one knew where I had been for almost two years. It truly felt as if this were no longer my home – but I had nowhere else to go.

When I was first discharged from the service, I was angry. I could not help but remember what I had done and what had been done to me, not only in 'Nam but also upon returning home. I knew I would have to take my anger and sense of betrayal to the grave with me. There was no way I was going to show any weakness or emotions. Even when surrounded by family and being with my wife, I felt alone. I could not imagine that any others were feeling what I was feeling, or that others had experienced all that I had.

I had a burning desire to tell someone how I felt, but these emotions were unacceptable to me. I did not feel like the man I should be. I was 21 now, and a man in every way. My father had taught me well about what it meant to be a man: it was to be stoic and to show no emotion. In his eyes and, ultimately, my own, showing emotions was a weakness.

Just as I had hated the world that I found when I went to war, I also hated the world that I found when I got "home." I knew I was a different man than I was when I left, but the world that I had left behind had changed, as well. I spent very little time in my hometown, because there was nothing for me there anymore. Several of my classmates had avoided the war. I wanted nothing to do with them, and most of them didn't want anything to do with me, either. No one looked at me the same. I was just another crazy Vietnam vet. It is interesting that it has taken me over thirty years to discover who else from my hometown had served in 'Nam. Like me, they, kept it a secret for most of their lives.

One friend in particular comes to mind. We called ourselves cousins, because we had spent so much time together as we grew up When he got to 'Nam, he got really scared. His parents were wealthy, and figured a way to get him home, allegedly because "they needed him for farming." This was an act of cowardice that I have never forgiven. Whenever someone comes home, someone else has to replace him. Did the guy that replaced him die, get maimed, or is he living the kind of life that I am? I often wondered if it was only the poor who went to war. I think part of the reason I extended my tour twice was that I was afraid of what would happen to my replacement. I didn't want anyone else to die in my place. Carrying the ghosts of two men who died in my place was quite enough.

I did visit my local VA hospital after discharge, but not to address the anguish I was experiencing. I had messed up my knee at some point in 'Nam. I had no clue what had happened to my knee, but while I was in country, there was no room for pain. Sure, the knee hurt, but it was just something I felt I had to accept. Upon my return, however, I decided to let the government pay for treatment. It never occurred to me at the time to say anything about the emotional turmoil boiling inside. It had taken several months just to get them to look at my knee – so how much luck would I have had getting help for something they couldn't even see? Besides, at that time, they had had no clue what PTSD was, so who knows what they would have done to me. I do feel that they would not have believed me. At any rate, they finally determined that the problems I was having with the knee were service-connected, and that I was thus eligible for treatment. I had constantly heard horror stories about the VA; the consensus seemed to be that it was not a friendly place for a veteran of *any* war. I found this to be true, and after just this one taste of veterans' "benefits," I vowed never to have to go to the

VA again. They did not make me feel proud that I had served my country. To them, I was just "another damn vet."

I ran into my old best friend one time when he was home on leave. Before I came home, I told my brother to get rid of my guns. I did not want to touch a gun ever again. My friend, on the other hand, came home bragging about all the gooks he had shot, and all the situations in which he had been involved. He was so proud of what he had done, and had decided to stay in the military. I really did not want to be around him. There was something about him that scared me. He was not the same friend I had known when we were young, and for the next thirty years, the old friendship I had once cherished simply didn't exist.

I soon realized that I wanted nothing to do with *any* Vietnam veteran. If I found out that someone had been in the war, they were history as far as I was concerned. I would not even talk to Vietnam vets. I did not want to be reminded of the war. I was so afraid that a vet would say something that would trigger the memories that I wanted to stay right where they were, stuffed deep inside me. I hid my involvement in 'Nam by not shaving or getting a haircut for three years. I would rather look like a hippie or even a protester than look like a vet. The country that I had served made me feel ashamed of that service.

There is a rage still burning within many veterans from Vietnam and other wars. It does not matter whether the veteran enlisted or was drafted; the country does not hold them harmless. Most Americans are not upset about the millions of dollars made by individuals and corporations because of the war. I even read – but cannot verify – that LBJ's wife made money every time a helicopter crashed. The soldiers, who followed orders from officers, who in turn followed orders from Washington DC, came home to protestors who spat upon them and called them baby killers. Where was our parade? Where was our "thank you?" Where was our respect for having defended this country? There was only anger at those of us who served. No wonder there is a rage within us, a rage that leaves the public scared of us.

Even after returning home, I continued to smoke marijuana whenever possible. It had a very calming effect, and helped me stuff everything even deeper. That was about the time a cigarette rolling machine called the Laredo came out. While it was meant for hand--rolling cigarettes, I found it to be the best way to make joints that could be carried in my cigarette pack, since they looked just like regular cigarettes. I also became very dependent on alcohol. Sometimes, I would drink to the point of passing out, and my friends would need to carry me home. Surprisingly, neither drug had any serious effect on my studies. This was all self-medication. At that time, post traumatic stress disorder did not exist as a diagnosis. I knew I was a little crazy, but would not be locked up for it. I knew that I had the ability to do something with my life, but also knew the VA would be of no help. I had to cope any way I could.

Though I did not realize it for thirty years, my three brothers were afraid of me. They have told me that I seemed to have a chip on my shoulder that I wanted someone to knock off. I had a hair trigger temper, and it seemed that I was always looking for a fight. I was angry at the whole world, filled with rage at myself and the secrets I was forced to keep. I was so ashamed when I learned that my own brothers, whom I love dearly, had been afraid of me. Nevertheless, I kept my secrets for thirty years. I thought I was quite exceptional, the only one struggling to keep those secrets from everyone.

In those early years, I had many nightmares of all the things that happened in 'Nam. I do not remember any specific incidents for the first few years, but there was one time, four or five years after the war, that my wife found me hiding behind a clothes hamper. Another time, I jumped out of bed after a nightmare and literally got "rug burns" on my knees – from the wall. I don't remember what the dream was about, but my knees hurt for a long time.

I knew the war was still there within me, but I had my duty to my family. I needed to find a way to function and provide an income to give my family what it deserved. Luckily, my wife always worked, which gave me some leeway. With all the jobs and positions I held in thirty years, I needed that flexibility. Even so, the road back home was to be longer and more difficult than I could ever have imagined.

CHAPTER SIX

COPING WITH WORK

Work became my way of coping with the war. As I look back on my career, it is a wonder I lasted as long as I did. It must be the Norwegian in me. I learned very young how to work, and even as a child, understood the importance of work in supporting my family. Despite having such insight at an early age, the saga of my jobs as an adult almost sound like a soap opera. I will not bore you with everything about every job and position I have had, but will describe enough so that you will understand how PTSD affected my working life, even though I had no clue that anything was wrong with me most of the time.

Over the thirty-year period, I held ten different jobs and/or positions, the best of which I sabotaged. I was afraid of both success and of not being in control of every aspect of my life. I distrusted my superiors; actually, I did not trust anyone who was in a position of authority. I did not trust anyone in the organization. I had a hair-trigger temper. I was not a team player by any stretch of the imagination; I always needed to be in control, and wouldn't play the political games. I was also a perfectionist in most areas, and wanted everything done my way. Even though I was technically capable, I often found myself being fired or suddenly laid off. I knew I had a temper but thought that being a bastard was an inherent personality trait, and that there was nothing I could do about it. I lived mostly in my own head, not letting anyone get close enough to know the real me, not even my wife. My mood would swing wildly on a moment's notice. That kept people at a distance, and that is what I wanted. I could not trust and I could not be a friend. Above all, I still avoided all Vietnam Veterans. I wanted nothing to do with a vet.

I coped by throwing myself into my work. I went to college, but it took so long for the VA to start my GI Bill payments that we were forced to go on food stamps for a short time. That left me feeling ashamed that I could not provide for my family. Throughout college, Alice and I had to work, because the GI Bill and scholarships were not enough to cover all the costs, and neither set of parents was in a financial position to help. Nevertheless, I have to admit that I was a little competitive with my wife, and was determined to get my degree. Knowing all too well my high school record of accomplishment, my wife was genuinely worried that I would not make it in college. But I knew that I had to have options other than the military, and a degree was an essential requirement if I was to have other choices. I made it through college, receiving my four-year degree in three years, graduating in the top 10% of my accounting class.

I received my CPA (Certified Public Accountant) certificate after a few attempts, and purposely sought out jobs that would require that I work long hours. Better to spend my waking hours dealing with numbers and tax laws than dealing with people – even Alice. My first job was with a small CPA firm. The hours were long, and I liked most of the work. The only drawback (and it was a big one) was that the owner of the firm was a control freak like myself, so there was friction between us almost immediately. Pretty soon, little things that other people would have overlooked or just shrugged their shoulders and accepted started bothering me. I worked on company buy-outs, and my job was to maximize the tax benefit for my client while in effect screwing the other person. This seemed too much like war, the victim being the guy on the other side of the negotiating table from my client.

Our daughter was born in 1976, and I soon realized that, with the schedule I had taken on, I would be going to work before she woke in the mornings, and coming home after she was in bed. I really wanted to be more of a dad to her.

My performance review, when it finally came, was quite an awakening. When I had first joined the firm, I was told that if I did a good job for three years, I would be made a partner. During my review, however, my boss told me that I was doing a great job, and if I continued to work at that level for three *more* years, I would be a partner. It did not take me long to find another job, whereupon I told him to do something to himself that was physically impossible. To this date, he has not taken on partners, and probably never will.

My next job found me working at a university as part of the internal audit department. Although the benefits were great, the hours were strictly eight to five. Once again, I had a boss who was controlling. In addition, some of the people I audited threatened me, both professionally and physically. I took those threats very seriously, and had a hard time not responding in kind. With the rage that still simmered in me, I was afraid I would eventually lose it and "take the sucker out." It was time to move on.

My second position at the university was as senior accountant in the controller's office, easily the most boring job I have ever held. There were a few major projects during the year, but the rest of the time, it was just plain boring. I started to teach accounting again (I had done some teaching when I was with the CPA firm). This became a ridiculous endeavor. In the hundred feet between the accounting building and my office, it was necessary for me to forget all the accounting theory that I was teaching to my students, because that was not the way the university was run. Although the pay was good and I was in a position for advancement in central management, I just could not take the boredom. In addition, the office was very political, some of my superiors were idiots, and there were sexual scandals that I happened to walk into. I was told, in no uncertain terms, to keep my mouth shut. I started looking again.

My next job was as business manager of the Chemistry Department. This job fitted me much better, even though the move reduced my chance for central management positions. I was the fiscal manager and advisor to the faculty. This put me in charge. I spent long hours working and improving the system. I introduced computers into the department, including implementing a dedicated word processing system in the very early days of personal computers. The fact that I worked long hours and had control over my responsibility made this a very good job for me. As long as I kept everything working right, the department head and the faculty did not mess with me.

I then let my ambition take over, disregarding my control needs and my dislike of bureaucracies. A position had opened up for the controller at a major private university in Des Moines. I applied, and unfortunately, I got it. Although this was the highest position that I had ever held and I was being paid very well, the position was wracked with professional and personal pitfalls. My staff was very poorly paid, which meant that I could not surround myself with quality people. There was a lot of pettiness among the staff, and the worst rumor mill I have ever encountered. They had spent over $100,000.00 on a new computer software system that I was to install, but they really wanted it to look and act like the old one. I found this absurd, since that meant that I would have to "dumb down" the new software to the point that the additional power and features it offered were completely disabled.

The majority of the accounting staff did not like me. I am not sure of the reason, but it is a feeling I have experienced frequently throughout my career. I did not broadcast that I was a Vietnam veteran, but people have often seemed afraid of me, nonetheless. About the same time I was hired, they hired the vice president to

103

whom I reported. I was not apprised of his background, but it was obvious that he did not have much experience in college finances. He was also the type who had no concept of chain of command, and would call in my staff for advice without my knowledge. We did not get along from the beginning. The position kept me busy twelve to sixteen hours a day, seven days a week, and it took a twelve-pack of beer a day, just to calm me down enough to be civil to my family. It was a horrible working situation, and practically eliminated my home life.

I stuck it out for nine months, but it became obvious to me that the situation was not going to change. The VP told me that I was going to be fired in the near future, so I beat him to the punch and resigned, giving myself three months to find a new job. During that three-month period, I just didn't care. I went through the motions every day, but refused to work the long hours, seven days a week.

With the help of others in administration who liked me, I landed a job as audit director for a bank. It was a relief to leave the university. There were some people there whom I missed seeing every day and working with, but I just could not work for an idiot, and would not work with a staff that did not have any loyalty to me. Soon after I left, the VP was dismissed, and I received several copies of the campus paper that announced this event from my friends and supporters who were still there.

I'm sure you've heard the old saying, "out of the frying pan and into the fire." The phrase could well have been coined just to describe the next job in which I found myself. I was hired as the audit director of a bank. I did much better with the staff, who at least seemed to be respectful, but this was the first time that I had been placed in a cubicle work environment, which turned out to be a major problem for me. It was very difficult to cover my back in a cubicle, and being able to hear all the conversations going on in the room further increased my anxiety. My cubicle was against a window that looked out on a large foyer, leaving me feeling completely exposed. It was not a safe place, or so it seemed to me. It also took me very little time to figure out that many of the bank's major assets were worthless. Seeing that the bank's end was in sight anyway, I hit the job trail again.

It did not take me long to land the position of Vice-President for Business and Finance for a non-profit agency. The pay was lousy, but I thought it would be nice to work for an agency that helped people. However, things were not quite what they seemed on the surface, and for the first time, I discovered what it was like to be sexually harassed. The president of the agency was a female, and made it pretty clear what she wanted. If you knew me, you would know how funny this scenario was, as I am hardly the type who makes women swoon. At one point, I walked in on her and another employee having sex on the boardroom table. It was very hard to sit around that table again without the images coming to mind. The Vice-President for Fund-Raising was also aware of her inappropriate behavior, and also learned that the woman had been using agency funds inappropriately. The two of us went to the Board of Directors with this information, assuming they would want to eliminate the source of scandal. To our surprise, it was not long before we both showed up for work and were told to have our desks cleared out by the end of the day. They called it a layoff, but we knew better. You either play the game, or you lose. I lost, and found myself unemployed with no real job prospects. I learned a few years later that the director was arrested for embezzlement. I never found out what her sentence was, but it was surely poetic as well as legal justice.

It seemed that I was overqualified for every position available. It was frustrating, because all I really wanted was a job. Finally, there was a job opening working with research grants at the university where I had been before, and the supervisor was someone I had known and maintained contact with for years. He hired me because he knew I needed – and could do – the job. So after five years, I was back at the same university; my pay was just drastically lower. It was another of those jobs that took about two hours a day to complete, so once again, I was back to the boredom.

About this time, I became heavily involved in the Boy Scouts. I had started as a troop leader before I left the university the first time, but now it became a passion. When I was not working at the job, I was scouting. At one point, I camped eleven weeks in a row.

The good thing about my position at the university was that I got along very well with my superiors. These were people that I had known for years, but had never worked for directly. I made significant improvements to much of the computer system, earning for me their trust and loyalty, which was to be of vital importance to me in the near future.

My bosses knew that I had taken about a 50% pay cut when I accepted this position, so it was no surprise to them that I continued to look for a better position at the university, which did eventually open up.

The position was in a veterinary hospital affiliated with the University, replacing the prior hospital administrator, who had been fired for sexual harassment. But I had to fight for the position. I was one of the finalists, but they offered it to a woman who currently worked in internal audit. Knowing her – and that her background did not qualify her for the job, I filed a complaint. She had been selected because of the sexual harassment problem. After I filed the complaint, the university's attorney had it in for me. He started to have meetings to ascertain *my* qualifications for the position. He called in my two direct supervisors, who were shocked that the only real question they were asked was, "Tell me what is wrong with Helle." Of course, they told me about this, and how stunned they were at his tactics. It only took one contact from my lawyer, to whom I am married, to resolve the issue, leaving the university no choice but to give me the position. The lawyer and the hospital director were ultimately terminated.

I found the place to be in a total mess and, like always, I soon found myself installing new computer software. They hired a new hospital director, who was excellent to work with. The finances of the hospital were turned around, leaving the hospital in a position to add several staff members and purchase new equipment. This was a lot of fun, even though it took a lot of time.

Administration at the university was a farce. It would take a whole book to describe the level of their ineptitude. The main players were the faculty, and the pervasive mentality was that each professor was allowed to do whatever they wanted, whenever they wanted. Though the university is known for its rules, it did not seem to matter if the faculty broke those rules or did things that were technically illegal. Such antics were excused as exercises in academic freedom. However, when running an organization that relies on user fees to pay the staff, such a *laissez-faire* attitude made it extremely difficult. Many of the faculty disliked me very much, and the feeling was mutual. Regardless of what some people did, no one could touch them because they were tenured. During my time there, the university awarded tenure to several professors who were the source of many problems to the hospital administration. The fact that some did not like me did not worry me much, so long as the hospital director knew and approved of what I was doing.

After two years in that position, I started to have real problems with my PTSD. I will discuss the details of this later, but I was in a hospital for over eight months during those two years. The director – whose father also suffered from PTSD – supported me.

Sometime in the time period between 2000 and 2001, I publicly lost my temper with an employee. We had a problem that I thought had been solved via mediation among the employee, the faculty and myself. I had found a workable solution that the faculty supported, and the employee was told how we wanted this job done. In spite of the instructions she was given, the employee continued to do it her own way, while I was demoted because of the situation. Although I acknowledge that losing my temper verbally was not appropriate, it was something that other members of the faculty did on a daily basis. For some reason, losing *my* temper was worse, and I think it had something to do with the staff being afraid of me.

During that time, the relationships with my staff changed. In June of 2000, I was called in by the campus police. I assumed it had something to do with some stolen deliveries. Instead of discussing the robbery, I found myself in a small room with two detectives. They asked if I had PTSD and I told them I did. They told me that they received a number of complaints where other staff members were concerned for their own well being, since I had been allegedly been exhibiting frightening behavior, such as coming to work dressed in a military uniform and a flack jacket. They did not charge me with anything at the time. Whether I was, in fact, acting strangely, I cannot honestly remember, but I certainly did not believe so at the time.

The detectives would not disclose the names of the people who complained, but did say they had nine complaints. They said their report was considered intelligence and not part of my public record, but it would be available to other police agencies. This left me in an indefensible situation. I was not able to confront my accusers, but they were maintaining the file on me for their use and the use of any police agency that asked for it. If I had known what they were doing, I would have had my attorney with me, because their accusations were – to the best of my knowledge – unfounded, and the apparent "trap" they had set for me was very inappropriate. But these were campus cops who were not all that intelligent. My biggest concern to this date is wondering what federal agencies have that file now — but perhaps that is a little paranoia kicking in.

If they actually had nine complaints, that was a significant portion of my staff at the time. It was extremely difficult to go to work, knowing that the majority of my staff was afraid of me, and that a number of the faculty disliked me because of my job. There were only a couple of employees that I could trust, one of whom, as it turned out, was a Vietnam veteran like me.

It is hard to explain the feelings that were going through me. The things that they were accusing me of were, I felt certain, totally unfounded. I actually thought that, as a boss, I was very easygoing. I let many things go by that I could have used to harm an employee's career. I did not expect or want to be in a position where everyone had to call me sir. I hated that. And I tried to get employee, input even though sometimes I would do things my own way anyway. I have worked for people who were real bastards, and I tried hard not to be like them. However, these employees had their little "cliques" and it was not beneath them to gossip. So any flaw I showed became exponentially increased by the time it made it through the gossip mill. I was – in their eyes, at least – the crazy Vietnam veteran again.

My supervision responsibilities dropped from over 30 people to five. The director was afraid of the staff filing lawsuits. A big complication in this came about in 2002 when the director left, and was replaced by a temporary hospital director with no administrative experience. She started working directly with my staff, leaving me out of decision-making. I do not feel that she disliked me; she just did not know how to manage. I had two employees who were unwilling or unable to do their jobs the way I wanted them done.

One employee, with whom I had thought I had a good relationship, turned against me. She filed a complaint with the new management, charging me with many wrongdoings. She would attack me verbally, and was very insubordinate. Even with all this happening, they tied my hands, leaving me powerless to do anything about the situation. The other employee was also insubordinate, and inept as well, giving rise to a number of complaints from both faculty and staff. There were even complaints coming from the dean's office.

With all this happening, I was reaching my breaking point. In October 2002, my therapists were recommending that I get out of the job because of the effects of the stress on my PTSD problem. I fought them because I was stubborn and had a very strong work ethic. Although I had often been suicidal in the past, I was now becoming more homicidal every day. I think I really wanted to kill the man who raped me, but had no clue as to where he was. I dreamed of killing him. Since he was not available for me to kill, I started to generalize and displace that rage. I wanted so much for someone – anyone – to say something wrong or touch me from behind so I could hurt them. The worst part was that at those times, I would remember what had gone through my mind before, when I had been in a firefight: Nothing. I had been functioning totally on instinct. I was so afraid of getting into that zone, and maybe hurting or even killing someone without realizing it.

In January of 2003, I was really losing it, so my psychiatrist at the VA forced me to quit my job for my own – and my fellow workers' – good. The day after I left, I applied for disability pay from work and the VA. I no longer had a choice. I had realized that I could not work any more and would probably not be able to work for the rest of my life.

I am not suicidal or homicidal at this time, but the drugs that keep me on the "straight and narrow" also keep me in something of a daze. I can only work from my safe place at home, and even then, I can only concentrate on any one project for a short period of time.

It is taking me a long time to accept the fact that I am totally disabled. Work defined me as a person. I took a lot of pride in my work and what I was able to accomplish. I know that what I had built up over ten years at the hospital will be flushed in a few short years, if my recovery takes that long.

The hardest part for me to accept about my last job was that I was basically thrown out like garbage, both from central administration and from the hospital as a whole. It did not seem to matter what I had or hadn't done. Had I left for another job or retired, I would have been given a going away party and a small statue they call the "gentle doctor." Instead, I was told to stay away from the hospital. Overnight, I changed from a main part of administration to a disposable object, just like a piece of trash. That was a major source of stress for me, because I thought I had a few friends there. As it turned out, there had actually been very few people who respected me or who would be friends with me. I was alone again.

But I knew I had to move on, and I am trying, to this day, to do so.

CHAPTER SEVEN

COPING WITH FAMILY

The title of this chapter should really be "How my family coped with me." With the problems and behaviors I have exhibited for the last six years (or maybe the last thirty), I am surprised that I still have a family. I know that my wife's recollection of some of this chapter is different from mine, but this is my book.

Even before I returned from Vietnam, I was trying to tell Alice that she should leave me and find someone who could give her a better life. I loved her dearly, but I had realized that, for seventeen months in Vietnam, I had been trying to get myself killed. I do not know why I came home on leave to marry her, except for fact that I loved her deeply and was filled with passion for her. I did not want to leave her, but somehow knew that her life would be better if she spent it with a "normal" person.

I mentioned in an earlier chapter that as far as Alice and my extended family knew, I had been trained in the Army as a clerk. All my letters home told them I was doing just that and nothing more. While Alice was going to college, I wrote a letter to one of her roommate's friends, asking if I should let Alice know everything that was happening. Her advice was not to tell her. So I kept everybody in the dark, or so I thought. A few years ago, I found out that I had inadvertently told Alice a few things in my letters that gave hints as to what I was really going through.

At Fort Lee after I got back from 'Nam, I really expected Alice to be a subservient little wife and follow my every wish. She did go with me to drink and smoke dope with the 'Nam vets, but although she would drink a little, she would not let herself get high. One night, my 'Nam brothers and I decided that she needed to get drunk. Alice loved wine, so we got hold of some bootleg wine, and all made sure that her glass was always filled. She did not notice that I only drank a few beers, which was not normal for me. When Alice started feeling bad, the other wives found out what we had done, and were all pissed at the bunch of us. Alice was very upset with me because I knew what was happening, and actually encouraged it, rather than putting a stop to it. Needless to say, I was in the doghouse for a while, and she kept a better account of her alcohol intake at future parties. At the time, I had no idea how my actions could have – and *should* have – destroyed the trust she had in me.

I had come back from Vietnam suffering frequent nightmares, and filled with anger and with an extreme fear that my secrets would some day be known. I struggled to keep those secrets from everyone, even my wife. I would rarely say anything about 'Nam, and when I did, it was something trivial. It was over thirty years before Alice knew the real story about my service.

The rape I had been subjected to always haunted me, and probably always will. My deepest horror from that ordeal was that it left me haunted by the thought that I might be homosexual. After all, a real man would have stopped the attack, right? I wanted – no, *needed* – to do things that proved I was a real man. My wife took the brunt of my attempts to prove that I was a man, a *heterosexual* man. I was very sexually demanding. I also sought out other ways to prove, at least to myself, that I was a man. I cannot to this day define what a man should be, but have always been sure that I have fallen short of that elusive definition.

While we were still in college, Alice and I realized that we needed to go to a marriage counselor, and also ended up going to a special sexuality program. The "bad" part for me was that I married a very intelligent and stubborn woman, who, like me, had Norwegian blood. Thus the idea of my being in complete control of my household was absurd. Although Alice put up with my problems, she did not hold back on expressing her disapproval when she felt it was warranted. She did not like my smoking marijuana or drinking, and let me know it in no uncertain terms. Maybe she knew something I did not at the time.

For several years after college, we were into our careers. Alice was working with the Social Security Administration, and I had my job with a small CPA firm. We liked the college town, and wanted to stay there. My job was demanding and the hours were long, especially at tax time. I liked the work I was doing, and as I mentioned previously, the long hours were exactly what I wanted. My extra job teaching accounting part-time at the university kept me away even more, but I could justify it, since the future we hoped for required that we make more money.

I think it was 1975 when we purchased our first home, a small place with less than a thousand square feet. Nevertheless, it was a cozy little house for the two of us. In 1976, we were blessed with the opportunity to adopt our daughter, Lorna. At that time, we were very strong negative- population-growth advocates, and had planned to have one child and adopt another, thereby only replacing one of us in the world. We had not expected to adopt first, but jumped at the chance when it arose, and it was wonderful.

In 1978, Alice got pregnant. This meant we had to find a bigger place, since our little home only had two bedrooms. Alice had problems with pregnancies, so when we moved into our new house, she was the supervisor, leaving the actual physical work to myself and the few friends we were able to enlist. This was a much nicer

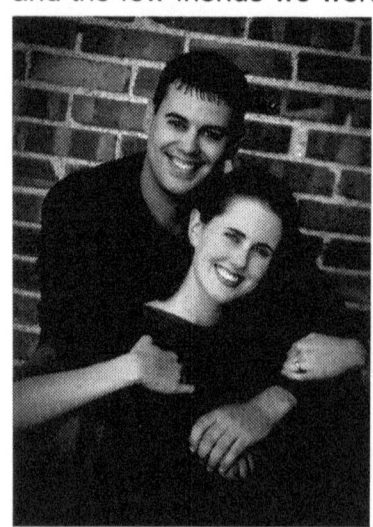

home, with sufficient room to raise a family. In May of 1979, we had our son, Sean. Now we had the perfect family.

The family was one of the most important things in life, a fact that I learned well with my upbringing. I tried my best to be a good father and husband to my family, but I was very moody, especially in the summer.

My daughter Lorna and her husband Patrick Looking back, I think that perhaps the heat, which had always been so oppressive in Vietnam, might have stirred up memories that I was able to keep buried away in the cooler months. But all too often, especially during the summers, my mood would change in a second, and I had no clue at the time why it happened. Even though I did have a bad temper, I never hurt my family. I was still a drinker, but had given up marijuana, mainly because possession at that time was a felony and being convicted of a felony would cost me my CPA certification. At any rate, when I remember what I was like to be around, I can certainly understand why some of our summer vacations were not my children's favorite memories.

We realized many dreams in our new house. When Alice was in her mid-thirties, she quit her government job and went to law school. Since we were living on only my salary, we sold the house and moved into a tiny town home to cut down our expenses. After she graduated, I got the job in Des Moines, so we moved the family

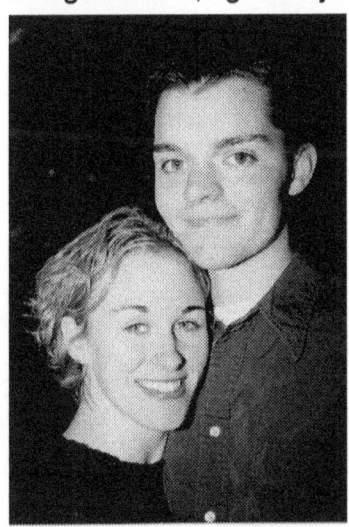

My son Sean and his wife Amanda

there. My children remember the Des Moines house as being home as they grew up.

We were never wealthy. People always assumed that, since I was a CPA and Alice was a lawyer, we must be rolling in the dough. However, I spent most of my career in the public sector. Although not as rewarding financially, I think that environment provided me with some sense of security that I needed. And Alice was never in law for the money. Her time with the family was very important for her. As with any profession, there is a relationship between the hours worked and the income received. Both of us chose a road that did not make us rich. We were not poor, but both of the children were working for their own spending money and "extra" things they wanted by the time they were 14. There was never a lot of extra money. But we did have what we thought was a functional family, which is easy to lose in the modern day world.

Alice graduated number one in her class, and started working for a firm in Des Moines, where she is now a partner. My daughter achieved her goal by getting a degree in psychology and sociology, with a minor in criminal justice. With an amazing amount of perseverance, she got into the police academy, and is now a senior police officer in Des Moines. At the time of this writing, she has recently married. Walking my daughter down the aisle had long been one of my dreams. My son, who has been married for two years now, just started his third year in law school, is currently ranked second in his class, and already has two job offers. He obviously takes after his mother.

This brief chapter, of course, does not cover every aspect of thirty-plus years of marriage. In most cases, we have led a very boring life. Even during the many times that I was very hard to live with, I just thought I was just another bastard, which it seems God made a lot of. (In the past I never did think much about God, but nevertheless we raised our children in the church.)

Throughout this entire time, I kept my secrets close to my heart, trying my best to appear normal. Although there were many signs of my PTSD during this period, I did not recognize that those signs were due to my war experiences.

When we raised our children, I did not have a gun in the house, and really did not want to even buy them play guns. My son, like many boys, eventually purchased a BB gun. Since he has grown up, he has become totally opposed to guns, and that does not really bother me. Of course, my daughter works with a gun at her side, and that *does* scare me. After 1998, I started almost obsessively accumulating guns, much to my wife's dismay. They give me a feeling of security, and are a part of my life that I cannot give up. Perhaps, one day...

When I fell apart in 1998, it was a shock to my entire family and to most people who had known me for a while. Remember, I had stuffed my feelings for so many years that I had become a master at it.

I realize that there are certain things in every person's life that should stay secret. However, there is a limit to how long a person can stuff feelings, emotions, and mental pictures, especially those borne of a horrible war, long over. Over the years, my subconscious has allowed me to remember many things that I would much prefer remain forgotten. I am aware that there are more such incidents that are only now starting to surface, and this awareness scares me to death. I feel as if I have remembered all the ugliness I desire, and then some. I do not want to know any more.

Even so, I realize that this knowledge holds the key to my recovery. I also now realize that I had to fall apart before I could begin to be put back together.

CHAPTER EIGHT

BREAKDOWN AND RECOVERY

THE BREAKDOWN

My world started to crumble in June 1998. I was in summer camp with the Boy Scouts from my troop. It was a normal camp morning: wet and muddy. I had the boys in my troop lined up for the morning flag ceremony, which we performed every morning before breakfast. Another adult Scouter had brought his toy cannon. While we were standing at attention, he shot that cannon off behind us. In the blink of an eye, I was face down in the mud. The boys thought it was funny, but in my head, it was not funny at all — I was scared to death. I went back, changed my clothes, and returned to help the boys have fun at camp. Unfortunately, that one incident caused the memories to come flooding back. I tried to stuff them inside me again, but it was a futile effort. I did not let any of the other adults know that something terribly wrong was happening in my head. I was not sure what was happening myself, so there was no way to explain it to anyone else. I just laughed off my reaction to the cannon, without trying to explain it. After that, the dreams were back, and the dark thoughts invaded my day. I had to have another adult take the boys to the rifle range, because even hearing the guns at a distance was causing me to have flashbacks. I stuck it out for the week, but I knew I was in trouble.

When I went home, I acted as if nothing had happened. I did not want anyone to know. John Wayne reared his head again, and I remembered the strength of my father. I still did not want to let my own wife know what had happened. I just thought I could get past this and life would be back to normal. Besides, how would I describe what was going through my head? I was feeling emotions that I could not describe and seeing images that I thought were long gone. There was just no way for me to understand these changes, much less, explain them to someone else.

In July, I realized that something was definitely happening to me, and whatever it was, it was not going away. I decided then to see the psychologist with my job's employee assistance program. He did not really understand everything I described to him, but he was the first person to mention PTSD to me. I could tell that what he was saying came from a fading memory of something he had read years ago. PTSD was something I had never heard of, and I had no clue how it related to my situation. I just thought I was just going crazy. The psychologist worked with my family physician to prescribe some drugs for me. In August, things seemed to settle down for me, so I stopped seeing the psychologist and threw away the medications. I hated the label of PTSD. Because of my upbringing, seeing a shrink, being labeled with a mental disorder, and taking those kinds of drugs caused me a tremendous internal conflict. I felt that it was a sign of weakness. I am not – and have never been – weak. All I wanted was to be a whole man, a good husband and father, and a good provider for my family. I was convinced that I could handle it all on my own.

That fall, I joined Vietnam Veterans of America (VVA). Why I joined, I had no idea. I was generally not a joiner, because I was so uneasy around people. I guess it seemed that I must at least try to be around others like myself. Though I started to attend most of their meetings, I never felt that I had much in common with the others in the group, except that we had all been in Vietnam. From what I could gather from the conversations, I doubt if any of them had PTSD, and I had some questions about whether some of them had even been in country at all. They seemed to be a bunch of egotistical men and women who liked to hear themselves talk, but I decided that I would give it some time. I had read the purpose of the organization on the web site, and it bore little similarity to what I was seeing at the meetings. Even though I was turned off by what I saw, I hoped that the group would eventually come around and try to meet the national standards. I had joined this group looking for some help from my brothers, but quickly learned that it would not to be forthcoming.

THE VET CENTER

In May 1999, I agreed to attend a meeting at the local vet center. I did not even know that the vet centers existed until then. Even if I had known about vet centers, I would have probably not gone to them. They were part of the VA system, and I still had hatred for and fear of the VA.

The people at the meeting were primarily a group of professionals from various vet centers, and representatives from veterans' organizations like mine. These professionals went around the room describing and interpreting patient actions and symptoms. I just sat on the edge listening. It seemed like they were stabbing me in my heart. Every time someone made a point about one of his or her patients or about an observed symptom, I just kept thinking, "That is me." It was horrifying. How could all these people know me? I wanted to run as far away as I could, but had nowhere to go. Tears were starting run down my face, and I was starting to shake.

I left the session. I could not bear to hear any more of this. I went to another room and cried for the first time since I was twelve. I was shaking uncontrollably. I was so scared. Was I like all these other vets? Was I too weak to handle my own problems? I was 49 years old, and this should not be happening at this time in my life. It had been over 30 years since the war. I had no clue what to do. A man soon followed me into that other room and when I saw him, I immediately tried to dry up the tears and get myself together. I did not want to be judged as a weak man. However, there was something different about this man. He just came over, put his arm around me, and told me to let it all out. I was in shock. He said he was Jerry, and he was a psychologist with this vet center. He told me he had been watching me, and knew that I had been affected by the discussion. He took me into his office and I told him that what they were saying hit too close to home. He made an appointment to see him within a few days. He asked me to promise not to "do anything" (meaning suicide) until we met. I promised and left for home. I was so glad to get away from that meeting.

I was extremely apprehensive during my first meeting with Jerry. As we talked, he seemed to understand me, and seemed to know exactly what was going on with me. I described my combat traumas, and nothing I was saying seemed to shock him.

I told him early on about the rape, but I insisted that it was not a problem for me. I had not told the psychologist at my work about the incident, nor had I told anyone else – not even my wife – because I was afraid of this memory. In fact Jerry was the first person I had ever told since it happened. For some reason, I felt I had to tell him; I think I was afraid it would come out accidentally, since I had come to realize for the first time that I was no longer in control. I wanted that incident taken off the table; I did not want him to be asking about it or making me talk about it. While I sat there in his office, Jerry called someone else to find out if it was possible that the sexual assault did not bother me. After he finished his conversation, I thought he believed what I had told him about it not being a problem I found out later he did not, but was letting me deal with the traumas as I could handle them.

I met with Jerry every two weeks. The summer of 1999 was extremely difficult, but with his help, I made it through. During that period the nightmares were very frequent, I would have flashbacks frequently, and at the worst possible times, even when driving my car. My panic attacks increased, scaring my wife, and I often had suicidal thoughts. Jerry referred me to a private psychiatrist, since I still did not want to go to the VA. Even though the vet center is part of the VA, there were no questions asked and no pressure to enter the VA system. The psychiatrist started me on some medications, which further helped me cope with the summer.

During our sessions, Jerry told me some of his story. Like me, he was a poor boy, and somehow got into the service underage at 16. He was in the armored division, and spent two years in Vietnam. He had seen comrades killed. He also had been shot in both legs. I could not understand why he seemed so interested in me. One day, he looked me in the eyes and said, "I don't think I could have survived what you did." At first I didn't know whether to believe him or not, but the look in his eyes told me that he was telling me the truth. He was a man who had seen much more combat, and was combat wounded. I was just in shock.

I sometimes called Jerry a bastard because he made me talk about things I did not want to discuss. Since things settled down for me in the fall, he started telling me how anniversaries of traumatic events could be difficult for some people, something I had not heard of before. Since my summers seemed to be the worst time of the year, he suspected that the events that still haunted me had probably happened during the summer. We discussed the events that had happened, but also talked about the upcoming summer, and ways to prepare myself for the anniversaries, even though I could not consciously remember the dates.

Jerry talked – with my blessing – to my wife and both of my kids. He wanted them to know what had happened to their husband and dad. I had given him approval to talk to them about anything they wanted to know about me, except for the rape. That was something I was not willing to share with my family yet. In one of their discussions, my daughter told him, "We had a perfect life, and all of a sudden it's gone."

In the meantime, probably since before I started seeing Jerry, I unconsciously started to revert to the soldier that I had been thirty years earlier. I acquired an AR15, which is the closest rifle to the M16 that a civilian could buy. I started to spend a lot of time on eBay, searching for missing pieces. I acquired a jungle uniform, boonie cap, Vietnam combat boots, flak jacket, and helmet. There were other things I purchased to complete my uniform, without even realizing what I was doing. This was happening unconsciously. It was as if I was preparing for war again. Of course, I kept all this hidden from my wife. I knew she would not understand. Hell, *I* did not understand!

In November 1999, I experienced my first suicidal crisis. That year, I had decided to visit the Vietnam Memorial in Washington for the first time. My wife was going with me; she would not let me go by myself. On November 8th, I was part of a Veterans' Day ceremony at the Iowa Vietnam memorial as part of the VVA group. I had read the name of a high school friend on the wall, and laid the memorial wreath at the ceremony. The event had was very depressing to me. I went home that day, and found myself alone in the house. My depression grew deeper, and I was drinking heavily. Soon, I had my AR15, locked and loaded, and had it pressed against my head. I continued to play with the rifle, fingering the trigger while I continued to drink. I was in so much emotional pain that I wanted out. I had reached the point where I did not think I could take it any longer. The pain I felt is so hard to explain. It was as if all the memories were in my head at the same time, along with the emotions attached to them. I felt guilty for not having died in 'Nam and for not saving others who did die. I was panicking, and feeling as if nothing around me – and not even myself – was real (The shrinks call this dissociation.) It was as if the weight of the world was bearing down upon me, and I was keenly aware that one bullet would end all of this in a fraction of a second.

I think the one thing that kept me from pulling the trigger that day was the memory of one incident where I saw a man shot in the head. It was as if I was out of my body, and could see the shot and his blood and brains covering the walls. I was hot with the realization that this was my home, but it also belonged to my wife. I just could not let her find me this way. I did not know how she could live in this house if every time she went downstairs, she would recall the same grotesque image I was remembering – except this would be an image of her husband after his last, desperate act. Somewhere deep within, I found the strength to unload the rifle and put it away. Instead of suicide, I called Jerry (not many government employees will give you their home phone number). and told him what was

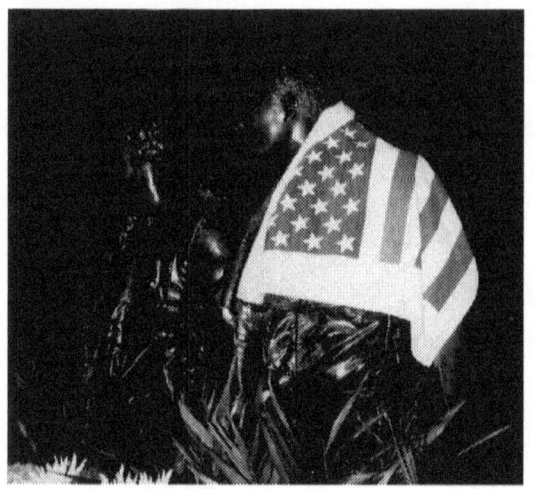

happening. He knew I was intoxicated, but he also knew that I was reaching out as I had never done before. I told him that I needed help, and asked him to find me the best program in the country. I did not care where it was. I just wanted to get past this. He agreed, and then made me promise I would not hurt myself. If I felt that way again, I was to go the emergency room. He cared, and that caring probably saved my life that time. I did not tell my wife about what had almost happened that day.

I survived the trip to the Wall in Washington. My original thoughts had been to take the .45 I had acquired and kill myself with it, close to my buddies whose names were on the Wall. But Alice flew with me to Washington, so that could not happen. I've often wondered if she knew more about my thoughts than I knew – or than she let on.

Being confronted with the reality of the Wall was much more difficult than I ever could have imagined. I had seen many pictures of it, but being there was so much more powerful. Except for my high school friend, I did not remember any names, and was not even sure of the dates. I sat on the benches around the Wall for what seemed like hours. Even then, it took me three visits to work up enough courage to actually go down and see it and touch many of the names. I had Alice with me to hold me and cry with me. The amazing phenomenon was when complete strangers, men and women, would come over and just give me a hug. These people knew what I was going through. I also learned then that I could actually hug another man– a concept that had always been foreign to me. It was just something I was taught: that men do not touch other men, except for a "manly" handshake. However, it seemed natural there to hug a brother who knew and shared my pain. Over and over, many of my brother veterans welcomed me home. It sounded so good to me. It was the welcome that we had so desperately needed, but that our country couldn't bring itself to give.

Much later, I found that I had two anniversaries in November, and no doubt these were the triggers for my suicidal crisis on Veterans' Day. First of all, it was in that month that my Dad had died. In 'Nam, it was when one of my men committed suicide. There were powerful emotions attached to each incident. These events, along with the Veterans' Day ceremony, had combined to plunge me into a very serious depression that day.

When I next saw Jerry, I found out that he had pulled many strings to get me into the program at the National Center for PTSD in Menlo Park, California. It was difficult because the vet center was the only place I had been receiving therapy, and there was no official VA file on me. I had not filed a claim for disability, because it still seemed too much like welfare to me, and I still had a very strong fear of the VA. The program in Menlo Park usually had a six-month waiting period, but Jerry was able to get me into it in two months. Even though this was what I asked for, I was scared to death. When

I got home, I told Alice about the program. She said that if that was what Jerry and I thought should be done, she was in favor of it.

I was lucky at work; there was no problem with my taking sick leave to attend the program. My son was studying in England at the time, and really thought he should come home when we told him I was going in. I convinced him that it would do no good, and that I would call him from time to time. At that time, I thought I would only be gone for six weeks.

A difficult part of the program was that I was required to be substance-free for thirty days prior to arriving. The drugs were easy, since I was no longer a user. However, giving up drinking was very hard. On the last day I could drink, I got together with several friends and drank excessively. It was as if I was drinking for the next six weeks.

THE NATIONAL CENTER FOR PTSD

In January 2000, I flew into Sacramento a few days early to my brother who lives there. When it came time for him to take me to Menlo Park, I was coming up with every excuse possible to avoid entering the program. I wanted to just go home and forget all this crap. My bother would not listen to me and, since I had no transportation, he did not leave me much choice but to go ahead and show up.

When Mick delivered me to the program, I was still trying to chicken out. They let him come in for a few minutes, and then told him he had to leave. I felt so alone and apprehensive about what was about to happen. It was at that point that it once again became obvious to me that I was no longer in control.

My initial reaction to the program was that it was much like being back in the military. The first order of business was a physical. I was glad that I had gotten used to female doctors, or in this case, a nurse. In addition to giving me a very thorough physical exam, she wanted to know everything about me and everyone in my family, which was a challenge in itself, given my memory problems. She had a nursing student there, who remained present throughout the examination. Although the student remained very professional, I was having some fears that I would have a "natural" reaction to being naked in the presence of a young woman. To my relief, the reaction never happened.

Once I was processed in, I was assigned to a four-man room. Since leaving the military, I had never been housed with men. I had serious reservations about living with other men in the same room. Luckily, there was only one other person in the room at that time. A nurse went through everything I had brought and confiscated a few things. It really surprised me when they took away my medications. They were not very happy that a private psychiatrist, rather than one affiliated with the VA, had prescribed my medications. I think I blew them away when I informed them that this was my first real interaction with the VA.

They got me to the VA psychiatrist very quickly. He kept some of the meds the same as I had been taking, but added some others, as well. He looked to me like he was about fourteen years old. It was hard to talk to him, as it was hard to believe that he was actually a psychiatrist. I discovered in short order that he was a good and caring man, and I saw him often since I was new to the VA.

My roommate was an ex-marine I called Big Mike. He was so tall that they had to bring in a special bed for him. Mike and I hit it off, even though we would argue every night about which branch of the service was best, Marines or Army. We soon grew comfortable in the knowledge that, if push came to shove, we would cover each other's back. Such was the bond that was so essential among fellow soldiers, but that I had never experienced while in country. We would take our sleep medications at night and would talk until the meds kicked in. It was funny, because we each would discover that on many occasions, one of us would be talking to ourselves while the other slept. Big Mike has remained a friend to this day.

The program kept us very busy. We had to be up at six a.m., and sometimes we were in classes until nine p.m. The food reminded us all of the military cooking, but it was enough to survive. One of the greatest experiences we had was that during weekend passes, we could go off-base and get some decent food. This could be as simple as having real eggs, as opposed to the powdered kind that had the consistency of jello (and less flavor).

I was assigned a "big brother," which is part of the program. For the first week, I could not walk anywhere on the compound without my big brother or someone else who had been there more than a week. Although my big brother was a nice person, he had his hands full taking care of himself. I spent most of my time with others. It did not really bother me, because I did not feel that I needed to be babysat. I actually felt sorry for my big brother, because he had a real problem with disassociation.

The program had a good-sized rules book. Although I was expected to read each page, I soon learned that the rules did not mean much. When I complained about one rule, one nurse told me, "That is the way people like you think." I really disliked this nurse for the rest of my stay, as I did not want to be lumped in with everyone else. I still had a job and a family, and that was more than most of the guys had. In my mind, that had to mean that I was not as sick as the rest of them.

One of the most difficult requirements was to have one-on-one conversations with other patients. It was hard enough just to be there and put up with a quasi-military operation. Now, I had to talk to a significant number of other veterans every week. Although we were not to discuss our traumas, just discussing our lives was difficult. These were people I had never met, yet I was telling them some very personal things about my life. I guess I did become closer to many of the other patients because of these talks. An Air Force veteran whom I met during one of these conversations is still a very good friend of mine.

Most of the sessions were on cognitive behavior. We learned a lot about how PTSD victims think and how we could gradually change that behavior. Some of it made sense, but a lot seemed ludicrous. In addition, some of the topics were taught repeatedly, to the point of being boring. We always knew that we could leave any time we wanted, but I was just stubborn enough to stick it out to the end. I then found out that I would have to be there for at least sixty days. Fortunately, my boss said to stay until they released me.

I was able to get out on weekends, but weekend passes had to be approved on the previous Monday. I spent several of my weekend passes with my brother. That was such a wonderful change. The first few weekends Mick and his wife Char treated me royally. The novelty of my presence eventually wore off, however, and it soon became "you know where it is." The advantage was that Char always washed my clothes, which was so much easier than fighting for time for the washer and dryer in the barracks. Most of the other weekends were spent interacting with other patients, which was one of the program's policies.

My wife was able to come down for a three-day weekend. We spent the weekend in Monterey, and it was great. I really hated seeing her leave. I was very homesick. On another weekend, my mom and stepdad from Iowa, as well as my sister and her husband from Minnesota, flew in to see me. Some of the other patients were amazed when they saw the four of them were in the day room. Too many of the other patients had family within an hour of the hospital that would not bother visiting. I learned about some of the guys' ruined marriages, and about children who did not want anything to do with their dads, and it just made me sick. A few of the men's parents had even severed their relationships, all because of behavior caused by traumas experienced when their sons were serving their country. Sometimes it seemed that the program was too little, too late.

However, seeing the other men's torn families made me thank God for the closeness of my own family, and the fact that my wife and children supported me. My whole extended family supported me, as did the few friends I had. God has blessed me.

Part of the process involved a tremendous amount of testing, most of which was computer based, and interviews by psychologists. One test had a question about whether I ever felt suicidal. I answered honestly and I was amazed at how quickly members of the staff came into the room and took me to another office. They questioned me intensely about my thoughts regarding suicide, and made me contract with them to tell them if I had suicidal thoughts while I was an inpatient. I agreed, but knew that those thoughts were not to be shared with the staff under any circumstances. I completed the testing, and was diagnosed with PTSD, not that it was a real surprise at that time.

The other part of the test was a GAF score. GAF stands for "Global Assessment of Functioning," and just as the name implies, it is a measurement of function. The higher your score, the better you will supposedly function in society. Several of my friends got theirs first, and tested in the 50's and 60's. Being the smart-ass that I am, I let them know that they had to be a lot sicker than me, but when I finally got my score, it was in the low 40's. I could not understand how I could have scored lower than did my friends. I had always thought that I was in better shape than most of the other veterans, and could not believe that I was that ill.

At some point in the program, I was assigned a little brother. The brother I was assigned did not want to accept any of the rules of the program. Since his behavior was my responsibility, we were immediately in conflict. I tried to keep my cool, and kept the staff notified of the problems I was having with him. As an additional source of stress, he had been assigned to my room. He had more anger in him than I have ever seen in anyone. It came to a head one day when we were to attend some kind of special ceremony. Our instructions were specific about the time we were to be there, but naturally, my little brother disappeared, and returned to the barracks by himself, which was a violation of the rules. On top of that, he started to attack me verbally, accusing me of lying to him about what he was allowed to do. He even threatened me physically. Being called a liar and being threatened was the last straw for me. As we argued, I picked up a chair and was ready to smash him with it and beat him with the pieces. I really wanted to kill him, but in my mind, I knew that if I did so, I would be expelled from the program and probably charged with assault. The conflict in my mind was tremendous. I put down the chair and removed myself from the situation, but realized that I was losing it big time. I had hit bottom, and found myself crying uncontrollably. Although the staff tried to resolve the situation, I was not able to think logically about anything. I asked them to give him to someone else as a little brother, and move one of us to another room.

They removed me from my room that night and put me in what the patients referred to as the "crazy room." This was a room where they watched everything I did with video cameras. I think it was actually to watch me for suicidal intent. That is when I really got to know a nurse named Anne. She was the instructor for one of the courses I was taking, but I had not had any contract with her outside the course. That night, she spent two hours talking to me. I felt so ashamed for my behavior, and especially for the amount of crying I had done. She was very patient and reassuring, and made me feel like I was still a man. She explained that I had hit the bottom, could now start to heal. Without her support, I think I would have left the program that night. She is still an angel to me.

The next day, I found out that my errant little brother had been expelled from the program. I also found out that Big Mike had backed me up with the rest of the population. Because of the support of Anne and Mike, I was able to complete the program. The psychiatrist put me on some more medications because of this latest incident. I had a couple of other little brothers during the rest of my stay in the program, but they were good guys, and didn't cause me the kind of grief I had gone through with the "little brother from hell."

One day, I was called into the director's office and had a discussion with several of the staff. They discussed the option of my going through a part of the program called "focus." I'd already had to discuss some of my traumas during the testing phase, but this "focus" program was an intense process that would require me to delve into these traumas with other brothers. I was not sure I wanted to do that. However, I accepted the invitation to go through the program, which added another thirty days to my stay.

I did not have a clear understanding of the program beyond the fact that I would have to work on my traumas. I had watched other guys going through it, though, and knew from watching them that it would be tough. In fact many of the guys refused to go through "focus," and many others were not invited because the staff thought that they were not ready for the program's intensity.

While going through the "focus" program, I was with two other brothers. There were two professionals in the room; one was the program's director. The first phase was to discuss what we were like before the war. Then we went into the war traumas we had experienced. Each of us had to pick three traumas to present. We were randomly picked to discuss our traumas, spending a half-day on them. We called that the "hot seat." And it was a very intensive time for all of us. There were many tears shed and many hugs. I picked my three traumas – all combat-related – and presented them when it was my turn. The work we did with each trauma was very arduous, and I was relieved when it seemed that the process was about to end.

As we were leaving, the director grabbed me and kept me in the room while everyone else left. He told me that I had another trauma that I needed to discuss. I do not know how he figured it out, but he basically described my rape. He told me that I would again be on the hot seat the next day, and that I would be required to discuss the rape. I was terrified at having to discuss my rape with my brothers, and of how they would react to what had happened to me. I was afraid of rejection. The next day, despite the fact that every fiber of my being was screaming for me to run away, I did show up for the session. Apprehension doesn't even begin to describe what I felt inside. I told my story with tears rolling down my face. I had a hard time even looking at my brothers. To my surprise and great relief, however, they did not reject me. They were supportive of me, and expressed sympathy that I had to go through that in the war. But I was still extremely nervous and scared, and after the session I spent considerable time pacing and smoking. I couldn't get over the fact that I had told my secret to other veterans, and I was inconsolable for a long time. Once I truly accepted the fact that my confession had not caused my brothers to reject me, however, I began to feel a little better.

After a brief time to decompress, I finally got to go home. My spirits were very high; I thought the 90 days had brought me to a place where I could let go of the past and live in the present. The director made me promise to tell my wife about the rape. I agreed to do so, but was very scared of letting go of that secret. The thought of going home and going back to work, however, thrilled me, as three months is a long time to be away from both.

RETURNING HOME

When I got home, I had one day with my wife. She and my daughter were to leave for England the next day to visit my son. I had already made the decision not to go, but with my extended stay in the hospital, I almost missed her. I took a week off to get used to being back in control of my time and myself again, and then went back to my job.

When I left the hospital in California, they sent me home with a thirty-day supply of the medications I was prescribed. I immediately called the VA hospital in Des Moines to schedule an appointment with the psychiatrist before my medications ran out. They told me that the psychiatrist could not see me for three months. I begged them to call the hospital in California and have them fax my prescriptions to them, so they could be filled until I could see someone. They told me it was impossible. They obviously didn't care what would happen to me if I went off my meds, and were absolutely unwilling to expend any energy for me. Part of the problem was that I was not "rated," having not filed a claim for disability with the VA, so I did not really exist to them.

Upon hitting this brick wall, I immediately filed a claim. Then I had to go to my family physician and beg her to prescribe my medications until the VA determined that I needed them and issued me an official prescription. I finally got my appointment with the VA, but instead of talking to a psychiatrist, I was assigned to a nurse practitioner. At least I was able to resume my therapy sessions with

Jerry. If not for him, I think I would have lost everything I had gained in the hospital.

Before I even got home, the VA was sending me bills for my hospitalization. My wife did not tell me about them because she knew I didn't need the additional hassle. I had read everything the VA sent me before I went, and not a word was mentioned about charges. This was just another VA surprise. I worked with one of my senators to resolve the situation. It would not be legal for businesses to suck you into a situation where no fees were mentioned until the service was rendered, so I couldn't understand why the VA thought it could get away with doing so. Even with the senator's help, it took months to get them to remove the charges.

It took me a long time to find the courage to tell my wife about the rape. This scared me more than any of the combat traumas did. When I finally told her, she just looked at me and said, "I knew there was more to that story." She was referring to a story I had been telling for years, that some guy tried to touch me, and that I had kicked him through a wall. Somehow, she knew that was not the whole story, but had been wise enough not to push me to open up about it until I was ready.

I had gotten back home at the end of March, and my summer anniversaries were soon coming upon me. That summer was worse than the prior year, and I was getting discouraged. I had spent 90 days in a VA hospital, and returned home, only to be screwed by my own VA. So far, I had not even seen a physician at the VA hospital. The nurse practitioner who was supposed to be taking care of my medication needs did not really want to hear how I was feeling. She tried to pull some therapy crap on me, for which she was obviously not qualified. I had to contact the director of the hospital and complain before I was given the opportunity to see a psychiatrist and a psychologist. The psychologist (at least I think she was a psychologist) was assigned to me because of the sexual trauma. That turned out to be another VA farce, as she spent very little time with me, and offered nothing in the way of therapy.

At least I was assigned a real psychiatrist who would really listen to me. At first, I did not know what to think of him, but have learned over the years that he really cares about his patients. When things are going okay for me, I see him every three months. There have been times when he was worried about me that I have seen him weekly. He has proved to me that, previous experiences to the contrary, some people in the VA really do care.

That summer was a very tough time for me, but with the help of Jerry, I got through the nightmares, flashbacks, and all the other emotions. The fall went fairly smoothly for me, although I was drinking heavily again, and fighting some strong emotions inside. Throughout that time, as always, I tried my best to put on the face that my family expected.

COMING TO TERMS WITH MY SEXUAL TRAUMA

My sexual trauma was in many ways worse than my combat trauma. People can understand and relate to the horrors of war, but rape is another matter altogether. As a small town boy, I did not know people would do this to other people. It was especially hard since I had to face my attacker daily.

While still in the army, I had to do everything possible to prove I was a man. I had become a super soldier. I passed the E-6 board three years before I was eligible, and when I turned that promotion down I was offered a promotion to Second Lieutenant. I was always willing to volunteer for any kind of duty. My need to prove my manhood continued even after I got out of the Army. I still felt guilty for "letting" the rape happen to me, and it remained a terrible secret that I really never wanted anyone to know.

At some point, Jerry got me involved with a male trauma group at the county's victim services department. Jerry admitted that he did not have much experience with male sexual trauma, and thought this group might be a better place to work on the problems that memories of the rape continued to cause me. There were only a few men in the group, and I did not have much in common with them. The other men had experienced sexual abuse as children. I was the only one who had been abused as an adult. It was hard to tell these strangers that I was 18 when I was raped. I felt that by that age that should have been able to prevent the incident. I was an adult, after all, not a helpless child. I was also afraid that someone would say something outside the group.

One of the group's facilitators was an ex-Marine who had been to 'Nam. He was tough on me, never letting me off the hook. He made me tell all about the rape and the other traumas I had experienced; regardless of how badly I wanted to keep silent. Even though he was tough on me, it was obvious that was because he really cared.

In January 2001, I went to the vet center for one of our regular sessions. Jerry knew immediately that I had been drinking prior to the session. We talked for a while, and then he got on the phone to someone. It took a few minutes, but then I realized that he was looking for a bed for me in a mental ward. Then I started getting scared. He found a bed in a local hospital, called my wife, and drove me there. He stayed there until my wife came to ensure that I would not run. I was not sure where I was going, but I knew I did not want to be there. As I was checked in, I realized that I was headed for a locked ward. I had never been locked up before, and it scared the hell out of me. Once I was in this ward I had no way to escape. I tried to figure a way out, but was unsuccessful. The psychologist at the hospital put me on more drugs, so instead of being suicidal, I was in even more of a drug-induced haze.

Over the next six months, I was locked up several more times. I was extremely suicidal. I kept trying to find ways to die without anyone knowing it was suicide. I wanted my family to collect all they had coming to them, and knew that the insurance company wouldn't pay if my death were self-inflicted. I felt they would be better off without me in their lives, and that the money would do my family more good than I ever could.

My panic attacks increased in frequency and severity. I remember coming home one day before my wife. When she got home, she opened the garage door and found me sitting at my workbench, cutting on myself with a hunting knife. I was so ashamed, but the physical pain was much easier to take than the mental pain, and served to distract me from it.

One of the last times I was in the lock-up ward was just before my son got married. I knew I was in a crisis situation, but there was no way I was going to miss my son's wedding. I just told them what they wanted to hear so they would let me go.

At one point I even made an agreement with one of our neighbors that if Alice were not at home when I was having a bad day, they would take me to the hospital. They did have to do that once. They never asked any questions, just took me where I needed to be.

Sometime in the spring of 2001, an event happened that I am trying my best to forget, because of the shame I brought on my family. I was arrested by the local police in a prostitution sting. I was handcuffed and searched, my car was impounded, and they took me to jail in the paddy wagon. What made this worse was that my daughter is a police officer. The jailers knew who I was and she was called in from patrol. This was one of the most shameful incidents of my life – having to face my own daughter in handcuffs, and knowing she knew why I was there. I think the jailers gave me better than normal treatment because they knew my daughter and me. Later, I had to face my wife, who had arranged my bail. I could not explain my actions, other than to try to make her believe that they had nothing to do with my love for her or any lack of sexual satisfaction at home. At that time, I figured this would be something she could not forgive, and that we would soon be divorced.

That night, Jerry came to our house. It is still amazing to me that a government employee was willing to help, long after his official day was done. It was at this time that I told my daughter about the rape. Jerry helped us work through it by explaining that, because of the rape, I had a powerful need to prove I was a man. He was so much help. Even so, I kept my distance from my wife for a while, because I did not know how she really felt about this incident. My daughter kept her distance from me as well, and I figured that she would never forgive me for what I had done to her mom.

My wife insisted that we go visit my son in college and tell him everything. This horrified me. I was supposed to be the male role model for my son, and I had failed. Yet when I told my son the story of what had happened in 'Nam and my arrest, he just looked at me and said, "You know, Dad, this makes a lot of things make more sense." He has never shown any signs of rejection.

During this time, I was constantly afraid. My nightmares scared my wife. I panicked often, unable to control the rush of emotions. I would isolate. On a few occasions, Alice would find me beating my head against the wall; again, the physical pain was easier to take than the mental pain. My psychologist gave me a small amount of Valium that I could take when I experienced a panic attack. I tried my best to get my wife to leave me. I began to drink very heavily. Above all, I was very suicidal; I just wanted the pain to stop. I knew

I was spiraling rapidly downward, but I could not describe what was happening to me to anybody.

The summer of 2001 was rougher than the year before. I struggled, but with Jerry's help I persevered. I was unsettled inside; the monsters kept getting stronger. In the fall, I lost my temper with an employee, and was demoted. I had several co-workers file a complaint about me to the police; they were afraid of me. They were afraid for themselves. It again felt like the world was crashing in on me. But I was a man, so I struggled through the nightmares, flashbacks, panic attacks, and the severe depressions. Despite my demotion, I felt I was doing ok.

One night's meeting of my sexual trauma support group was especially tough, and I left the meeting very upset. I stopped and bought three large cans of beer and drank them while driving home. My wife was gone that evening, so there was nobody with whom I could talk. Then I thought of the friend I had made while I was in California. Although he did not know my whole story, we had been talking regularly since I left California, supporting each other. When one would slip, the other would pick him up. He was my buddy. So I called him – and I told him about the rape. About a week later, I received a letter from him. In that letter, he basically said not to ever again call him, write him, or come out and see him. His rejection was total and complete. In 'Nam, when you made a mistake, someone died. I felt I had made a huge mistake now, and I had lost another buddy. Although he was not dead, I had killed a friendship. I was devastated.

I went out and purchased a .45, because I wanted the pain to stop. I knew I would have a better chance of success with a .45 with hollow point bullets. I played it through my mind repeatedly. I did not want to do it in my home, because that would still be my wife's home after I was gone. I planned to head out into the woods so I could be by myself. I figured someone would grow suspicious about an apparently abandoned car, which would mean someone other than my wife would find me. I knew that Alice fully expected to come home one night and find me dead, but I was not going to let it happen that way. Still I wanted out. The pain was too great.

For some reason I decided to hang on a little longer, but the next six months were absolute hell for me. I spent a total of two weeks locked up in the hospital. My panic attacks came more often and were more serious, and I was mutilating myself. I was never sure what would bring back a rush of memories and emotions. Sometimes it was the heat, an overgrown area, or sounds and smells, and sometimes I just had no clue. I would either bang my head against a wall or cut on myself with a hunting knife. It seemed that the physical pain I inflicted on myself brought me a step back closer to reality, and away from all the emotional pain.

It was Jerry who rescued me again. He somehow knew that the rape was what was causing me to self-destruct. Now that the combat trauma was out, there was nothing to protect me from the sexual trauma. I was so scared, and trusted no one. I was making plans to disappear to Arkansas and live alone in the hills. I wanted to be totally alone. I wanted to desert my family. I wanted to run away from me.

Jerry found a program for sexual abuse at the VA hospital in Bay Pines, Florida. I know that he had to fight a lot of red tape with the VA to get me into the program. I had filed my claim, but at that point, the VA was not taking any responsibility, so I had to fight for help. The VA did not want to help me, insisting upon absolute proof that something could happen in a war zone – especially in an area other than in the front lines – that could have caused my PTSD. I thought they were damn fools; there were no rear lines. I wanted to be believed, and I wanted my government to acknowledge that I was harmed and that my life had been diminished because of the war. I did not blame my government, I just wanted them to believe me and offer me the help that I so desperately needed.

BAY PINES, FLORIDA

In August 2001, I went to Florida. When I left Iowa, I was not guaranteed a spot in the program. However, I had nothing else. If they were going to turn me down, they had to do it to my face. I was a dead man walking; my options were running out. I knew that I would not survive much longer at the rate I was going.

In Florida, I met Roger. Without even needing to interview me, he told me all about myself. He knew how I would act out in destructive ways. He also knew that I would isolate, and that I feared people. He scared me to death, because he *knew* me. I could not understand why I did the things I did, but *he* knew. I did not want anybody to know me that well. Hell, I did not know me that well. Although scared, I felt some relief that there were reasons behind my behaviors. I was not crazy; I was not mentally ill. I was reacting normally to an abnormal event. I saw immediately that Roger was not a threat. I somehow felt that he knew how to help me. His compassion, along with his professionalism, gave me some hope.

In the program, I learned so much about myself. I also met other men who were not afraid to admit to their rapes. Even though I was in the program, I still feared that truth about me. However, I met men who had served in the Marines, Air Force, Navy, Army, and Coast Guard – all of whom had been the victims of rape, and that it had screwed up their lives like it had mine. I started to feel that I was not alone.

The dormitory in which we stayed was co-ed. Although there were only men in my program, there were many people – both men and women – who were going through other programs or were there for medical treatment. I was scared that others would figure out for which program I was being hospitalized. However, at our first group meeting, I found out there were several guys I had been talking with who were in this program too. They also had a women's program there. There was one young woman named Linda with whom I got to talking, and I knew from the grapevine that she was in the women's sexual trauma program. One day, I received a letter from my niece, who had also been raped, and after reading it I was sitting in the day room in tears. Linda came over to console me, and for some reason, I trusted her. I told her why I was there, but hell, she already knew. We would spend hours discussing what had happened to us and how it was affecting our lives. It was amazing how similar we were. It was fantastic to be able to discuss this openly with both men and women.

I had been looking for my attacker for several years. I would (and still do) dream about grabbing him by the hair, slitting his throat, and looking at his eyes as he slowly dies. I want him to know who took his life, since he took mine. I know that the teaching of Jesus tells me to forgive this man. However, so far I have not been able to. I do not hate the Viet Cong, who were our bitter enemies, but I do hate my attacker. The lifetime effect of his act is worse than death. I would want him to know the hell I have lived and continue to live. Perhaps one day he will read this book, and know…

I was in the program in Florida for four months, and felt I had achieved a better understanding of myself. Roger was the only therapist who kept repeating, "I promise you nothing." At first, I thought, "Why am I here if the head of the program won't promise me anything from the program?" And in the beginning the group sessions were tough. Twice a week I found myself in a room full of men. They told their stories and discussed the problems they were having. I could not believe it; the room represented every branch of the military. Several marines in the groups were huge men that I would not want to meet in a dark alley. It was so hard to believe that they too had been raped, most in Vietnam, but others during their time at different duty stations. One Marine in particular kept saying that what he had learned in the program and in the group sessions was, "The healing is in the telling." The strength he showed me is why I can now tell the world everything in my books. He died of a heart attack while I was there, and it was like losing a best friend and a hero. This Marine taught me so much about myself.

A major part of the program was a five-week intensive group. In this program, we had to tell about our sexual traumas, and then discuss the normal behaviors of men like me. It was fun to watch Roger act out the normal behaviors– passive or aggressive. He wanted us to be in between the two extremes. He did not tell us how to heal, but only gave us the tools to understand what behaviors we could expect and how we could circumvent those situations. Roger was not telling us that the pain would disappear, but that we had the option to improve the quality of the rest of our lives.

When I got home, I had a new understanding of who I was and what my disorder might try to force me to do. I also understood that despite my disease I now had options in my life. I could find ways to control the feelings and do something different that was more socially acceptable, not to mention less personally destructive. It is no exaggeration to say that Roger had saved my life.

Not long after I graduated from the program, the VA system shut it down. Roger was forced out, and the remaining staff members were afraid of doing or saying anything that might cost them their jobs. I have tried to get someone in the VA to explain their justification for this action, but have only gotten the run-around. My senators and congressional representative would not get involved. The emails from a staff member started getting very aggressive. I had to back off because Roger had started a private practice, and my attempts to get real answers were hurting him.

I understand that they have since started a new program for men, but trying to find out anything about it has been an exercise in frustration. My interactions with a staff member were extremely negative. I therefore have no information about the similarities to, or differences from, the old program, but I do not know whether it can achieve the success rate of that program. I do pray for my brothers and I hope there is still real help for them. However, it is obvious that the military and the VA system do not want to admit that male rape occurs.

I made a promise to myself that I would not go to any hospital in 2002. Having spent over eight months in hospitals in the previous two years, I figured I had gotten all the help I could get. I did start going every two weeks to a private psychiatrist who understood all my traumas. Jerry left the vet center, and it took a while for me to gain any trust in his replacement. The primary treatment I was getting from the VA was the medications.

In 2002, I was getting very tired of waiting for a decision on my VA claim. It had been two years since I first filed, and I had not heard a word. I decided that I had to get my senators involved to force the VA to make some kind of decision. They finally came through with their decision, and rated me at 70% disabled. My service officer told me he could get me 100%, but I wanted to work. I was not ready to go out on disability at that time. I still thought I could make it.

CHAPTER NINE

DISABILITY

I did stay out of hospitals in 2002. Although I was stubborn enough to achieve my goal, it was not the best thing I could have done for myself. Starting in October, I began having aggressive tendencies. I talked about them with my counselors, and more than one of them told me I should get out of the work situation. That was not an acceptable solution to me at the time, because my work defined me. I needed to work.

In January 2003, the aggressive tendencies became intense. Instead of being suicidal, I was becoming homicidal. That was a new feeling for me. I was waiting around for someone to say something or touch me so I could hurt them. I did not care who did it; I just wanted to hurt someone, maybe even kill him or her. I remembered firefights in 'Nam and the fact that I did not think during the fighting. I was on autopilot then, with my sole purpose being to survive and kill the enemy. Now, as I found myself re-entering that frame of mind,

I was getting very scared that someone might enter my "kill zone" without realizing it. I did not want to kill again.

Sometime in January, I was really losing it. Alice took me to the local hospital, but they were full. Someone checked with the VA in Knoxsville, Iowa and discovered that there were beds available there. The last place I wanted to be in was a VA lock-up ward. I tried to back out, but the people at the emergency room said I could voluntarily go or they would get a judge to commit me. That was not much of a choice. They even made me take the hour or so trip in an ambulance. So in the middle of the night, I was being strip searched, and most of my belongings were taken away. I had to talk to some kind of professional, and then start wearing some very sorry looking pajamas. The next day, I talked my way out of the ward. After being in so many institutions, I knew what they want to hear, and fed it to them.

It was also in January that my VA psychiatrist wrote a letter saying I should not work. I finally gave up and filed for disability from work as well as full disability from the VA. In 90 days, I received my full disability from work. The VA has determined that I am 100% disabled due to being unemployable.

Although leaving my job was very beneficial to me because it reduced a major stressor in my life, being on total disability at fifty-three did depress me. It felt like a major defeat. It depressed me because of the work ethic I learned as a young man. I could get by on the disability pay, but that seemed like welfare to me, and I am opposed to welfare. Physically, I was fine, so it hurt that I could not work with people anymore. I do not expect this to change for the rest of my life. I am, therefore, forced to redefine my life.

WHAT NOW

Now they tell me that this is a good as it gets. The nightmares still haunt my nights. The flashbacks are still there. I am afraid, especially in crowds, and I still have panic attacks. I still have trouble over the summer because of all the anniversaries of my traumas. The heat of the summer does not help. Most times, I have no clue what triggers the symptoms. I have a hard time trusting anyone. None of this will ever change. I will never be that 18-year-old boy who went to Vietnam. However, I am coping. I know that I will be on medications for the rest of my life. I know I will need counseling. I cannot do it on my own. I am a step away from death, from running away, from hurting those around me.

But I refuse to give up. I will find my place in this world, I will find meaning to my life, and I will contribute to society.

I will be a man.

CHAPTER TEN

LOOKING TO THE FUTURE

For so many veterans, the battles continue for a lifetime. Whether their wounds are physical, mental or both – these men and women are the heroes of our wars, and should be treated that way. They are not now. I sincerely believe that every veteran who is disabled with PTSD should get the Purple Heart. The wounds of PTSD are deep, and most of us will die of those wounds.

My life is not concluded yet. With any luck, I have 20 or 30 more years ahead of me. These years need to be lived. I want to be as "normal" as possible. It is very hard to define what is normal, but I am still trying.

The philosophical question each of us must ask is how we can live those years with meaning. I get emails daily with stories that rip my heart out. I thought I was tough, but I hurt so much for my brothers and sisters. It is a hurt that I want to do something about.

I also ache for the things I see happening in this world that make me see my time in the service and in the war as wasted time. It seems to this farm boy that the more young people have to fight for our freedoms, the more will be needed to continue the fighting. I am perplexed at this point in my life, wondering whether we are fighting for the freedom of our country, or for some obscure reason that I cannot comprehend. I am not a political person, but there is something today that increases my fear. I fear for my own children, but also all the other children of this country. Will they enjoy a "normal" life, or will they be facing a world that will leave them like me? I do not want any of our children to live through the hell of PTSD. I pray for all children. One of my counselors defined childhood as age twenty-five and below. It was his theory that we are still developing in our early twenties and that certain experiences will have a more significant impact on our lives during this period.

MY MISSION

Calling something my mission sounds a little strange to me, but I have been told this by so many people I have come to accept it. When I was forced to quit working in January 2000, I had no concept of what my life would or could be. I felt like a lost soul. My brother Mick kept telling me that when one door closes, God opens another, and that I just have to be open-minded enough to see what is being offered – and to have the guts to go through that door.

I do not know if it was God's intervention or just personal inspiration, but I now feel that it is my duty to be an advocate for trauma victims. My heart goes out to those who have experienced traumas, both in the military and in civilian life. Both are equally disabling. The person I call God is the God of my youth, and He is my higher power. I know brothers and sisters who have a different higher power. Whoever your higher power is, the devastation of PTSD is the same, and the reactions to the higher power are much the same.

As I mentioned previously, when I went to 'Nam, I had planned to go into the ministry. After less than two months in country, I decided that this was not the appropriate role for me. I had broken too many of my God's commandments to serve him as a minister. I even questioned the existence of God, since He was allowing all these horrible things to happen to both sides. I could not reconcile this with my religion. Why would God want over three million people to die?

Then one day, some thoughts came to me. I know my wife and son thought I was crazy, but I had to write down the thoughts that were going through my head before I forgot them. The following are the thoughts I had that day.

MY MISSION

Something happened

What it was I have no clue

No clue where it came from

But it has shown like a light

In my heart

I have been so afraid

Of the vengeful God of my youth

Knowing what I have done

The sins upon sins

I was doomed

But suddenly

I felt a shield around me

It kept me safe in 'Nam

It is still here

I was blind

But now I can see

This is the shield of God

He is protecting me

Not from myself

But from the world

God's demands are strong

He kept me safe

Not from my traumas

But from the failure

To serve

God has a mission for me

It is becoming clearer

The shield will help me

Stay on the right path

And help my bothers and sisters

God has forgiven

All that I have done

But I now know

He is not done with me yet

I must serve him

I am to serve my bothers and sisters

And perhaps, one day

Forgive myself.

I started my service to others with the website for my first book (www.ptsd-alliance.org/AWALKINHELL.htm). Although I set up the site to sell the book, the response from trauma victims was tremendous. I received so many emails, and I have made friends who are still friends to this day. I still receive emails almost every day from soldiers and those who love them. It is nice that they know they can call me anytime, 24 hours a day. I have received calls at odd hours. I have talked three veterans out of suicide. I am so glad to be there for them. It readily became apparent, however, that I could not accomplish my goals by myself.

In June 2003, I established an Iowa non-profit corporation to help me do this job. I called the corporation PTSD Alliance. I have transferred much of the information from the book site to the new site (www.ptsd-alliance.org). Even though I am still selling the first book, most of the profits are being used to help maintain the alliance site. After four months the IRS granted the corporation the 501(c) 3 designation. This will allow us to obtain funding through donations and grants, so I can make this a national alliance.

I want to develop an alliance of sources throughout the web that will bring veterans' sites, trauma sites, professional sites, and other related sites together to meet the needs of trauma victims all over the country.

I also want to develop an alliance of volunteers (and professionals) who can work with vets in their area by listening to them and helping them get to the resources they need. This will give victims options they didn't know they had. This organization will not charge for membership or use. There will be people who can listen

and understand, because they have experienced similar traumas. This can be accomplished with the total autonomy of – and privacy for – the victim. We currently

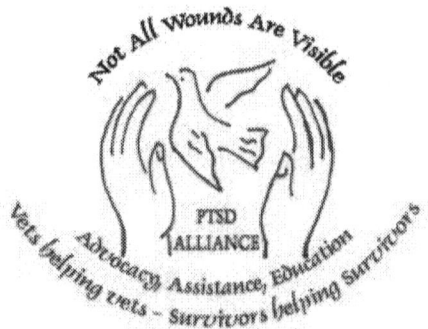

have over 120 volunteers in 27 states and 7 foreign countries. Funding remains a critical issue.

Although I would like to see victims receive the proper medications and psychological treatment, this alliance will at least provide an initial step for them. The fear of the government and/or people with initials behind their names scares many veterans thus preventing them from improving their quality of life.

My God has given me the ability to write and speak. Will I become world famous? Probably not. But a few of my books will reach people and help them or educate them about PTSD. I am already writing a monthly newsletter, which is distributed free by email. I continually write editorials and letters to editors, a few of which have been published. Even as I finish this project, I am starting new book projects.

Finally, I give speeches on radio and television, as well as to a variety of groups. This is the most effective method for me to reach the public and many vets. I have found that most of the people I have talked to have no idea about PTSD. Some have written months later, telling me stories about people they knew or people in their family whom they now understand better.

God willing I will find other ways to reach victims and the public.

CURIOSITY

As I explained in the Foreword, I do not intend this book – or my efforts in general – to be political, even though some of my statements may sound like political statements. They are just some curious thoughts of one man.

We currently have young men and women fighting in Afghanistan and Iraq. These young people are willing to give their lives, and many have come back severely wounded. Even the soldiers who come home as I did may have received wounds that are not visible, and may not be visible for decades. It seems to me that since we are asking these young people to place their lives on the line for this country, we have a lifetime obligation to each of them. They all deserve the best quality of life possible.

We are currently in an environment where we are sending more and more soldiers into harm's way. The images of the war are whitewashed for public viewing. We hear about the numbers of fatalities – but what about the rest? How many of our young people are lying in hospitals with varying severity of wounds? How many young soldiers have already come home with the initial signs of PTSD, not knowing or understanding it? How many of these young people are literally human time bombs, as was I?

At the same time, there are cuts in the VA budget that are already affecting the ability of these young soldiers to get help. I am getting older, and I have lived a good life, overall. Will we allow these young people the opportunity to live a good life? It seems to my mind that even as we are creating new veterans, we are cutting the help out from under their feet. As I remember, it took the VA ten years to admit to the Gulf War Syndrome. During those ten years, many veterans had to suffer. Why did it take ten years, and why didn't the VA take care of these soldiers, even without knowing why so many of them were getting sick? It does not make sense to me.

The term "patriotism" seems of late to just mean waving flags on special occasions, and paying lip service to our fighting men and women during the time that an official war is being fought. Most of the population has never been in harm's way. I am glad that they have not had to see the worst of the world, but I pray that they learn to have some compassion for those who have been willing to fight for the freedoms we all enjoy.

The events that I was a part of in Vietnam do not constitute much of a war story. I hear much worse stories from the vets I talk to and some of the books I have read. However, the quantity of the traumas is not the major factor. It is the effect that these traumas have on a person that matters. People seem to think that a person had to be in combat every day to have experienced trauma and suffered from problems as a result. In reality it only takes one event to shatter a life, and it can happen to anyone at any time.

I read lots of differing theories as to why some people are never bothered by the war, while others end up like me. I am not convinced that anyone in the psychiatric community really knows the answers. I think that is why society ignores people like me. They are frightened of that which they cannot explain, and turn away, rather than face the discomfort.

I am so amazed that there is no public outcry about spending another ninety million on a war that was declared to have been won months ago. Moreover, at the same time, the VA is cutting services and closing hospitals around the country. There are so many needs here at home, and I cannot comprehend why we can spend millions fixing a country we just blew apart, when our own people are on the street and going hungry.

I have given a few lectures around Iowa, and a few on radio stations around the country. However, I am left with a feeling that I cannot shake: that people do not want to hear about veterans. We live in such a wonderful country that most of us do not have to see the dark side of the world. People do not want to hear from those of us who *have* seen the worlds – and our own – dark side.

I am reminded of the few chess games I played and lost years ago. The front row consisted of the pawns. When I lost a pawn, it really did not hurt me much. But when I started losing the knights and other pieces, it became serious. As a non-commissioned soldier, I feel like I was a pawn in a political game I didn't – and still do not – understand. Now that I am not part of the military, I feel like a pawn that has been tossed aside. We are a disposable society, but I hope we do not just dispose of our young people, who are brave enough to defend our peace with their own lives. Even if we don't agree with the reasons they are doing so, we owe these young people our support, for they have gone where their duty has sent them, and performed as was expected of them.

Someone recently said, "They are over there fighting, instead of fighting here on our own soil." This keeps us safer here and allows us freedoms that we do not even think about, much less acknowledge. With our young men and women being placed in harm's way, every day should be Veterans' Day.

WORKING WITH THE VA

I have told my story, but there is more I wish to do. I also want to give my veteran friends some advice from my perspective on how to deal with the VA. This huge bureaucratic organization too often is itself a barrier to the vet seeking the help that the organization is supposedly structured to provide. I am sure this is true of other governmental organizations that exist to help civilian victims. It is my understanding that most health insurance policies do not cover mental health treatment. This leaves most of us to rely on the dwindling resources of governmental agencies.

Whether you are a veteran or not, this chapter has some critical advice for you. The public in general does not know much about PTSD or PTSS (Post Traumatic Stress Syndrome), and it is not a priority for them. They need to understand that for one suffering from these diseases, just surviving each day *is* a priority. People need to know how hard it can be for a victim to get professional help.

As we see state budgets cut, many of the cuts are coming out of mental health facilities and support. This is happening at the national level too. VA facilities are being closed down, even as we are increasing the number of new veterans who will need their services. In small population states like Iowa, veterans are going to have to travel further for help. Many of these veterans cannot afford the trip, or may not even have the means to make the trip. These changes will further isolate victims of PTSD and PTSS.

Gregory A. Helle

BE YOUR OWN BEST ADVOCATE

The best piece of advice I can give anyone, whether you are seeking help in your community, through your insurance company, or the VA, is very simple but very difficult: **BE YOUR OWN BEST ADVOCATE.** There are people in your community who are very willing to help you and advocate for you, but they have to know you exist. There are hundreds of good websites as well that provide information on PTSD and PTSS. There is some benefit to understanding your disease, but information by itself is not enough. The information you need to gather is what your community and/or state can do to help you. Check your health insurance and determine if there is any mental health coverage.

Whatever happens, remember that you cannot go it alone. This is a disease that requires professional intervention.

If you are a veteran like me, you will find – if you haven't already – that working with the Department of Veterans Affairs is a struggle at best. This agency is supposed to take care of veterans who have proudly served their country, but – if we are to judge by their actions – it does not seem to want to help. In order to receive benefits, a veteran must convince the VA that the problem was service-connected. If one goes to court in this county, they are presumed innocent until proven guilty. The VA works under an entirely different set of rules. When a veteran files a claim, the VA considers the claim to be fabricated unless the veteran can prove that the events claimed actually happened, and that the veteran was a part of that incident. Regardless of the financial status of the veteran, this initial claim process could take several years. In the meantime, the veteran must seek other forms of charity. Many are on the streets begging.

If the VA rejects the claim, there is a long process of appeals that takes much more time and energy than many veterans can handle. Many feel that the design of the claim process is intended to make the veteran give up, thus saving the VA money. A personal claim I filed six months ago with a private insurance agency took only 90 working days. The VA is still working on the same claim. I have had to ask my senators and congressional representative to attempt to find out why my claim sat on somebody's desk for six months without any action. Now that I am on full disability from my job, I have lost a considerable amount of my prior earnings. If not for the fact that I have a working wife, I do not know where I would be.

The claim process for the VA is separate from the medical and psychological duties of the VA. I have met so many people working within the Veterans' Administration who really care. However, the hospitals and programs are tremendously understaffed. Many times, a vet who comes in for treatment will see a nurse or nurse practitioner, and may not even see a doctor. It can take six months to get a medical appointment. In the mental health section, a patient can only see a psychologist every six months, and a psychiatrist every ninety days. These people do care, but there is not enough funding to serve the veterans. To make matters worse, the current level of local mental health support is substandard. The new veterans are finding it very difficult to get appointments. They return from a war that the country backed, only to find that they are as expendable now as they were in the war, perhaps even more so.

Working with qualified psychologists helps us understand the destructive emotions we feel and how we can better cope with them. There is no escape, only coping. There is, however, hope. My life today is much better than it has been over the past six years. I will never be "normal," but I have hope that I can enjoy much of the rest of my life and enjoy my grandchildren when they join my world. I am lucky enough to be able to get the help of a private psychologist. As implied above, those who have to rely on VA psychologists may wait months between sessions, and too many of them see their lives destroyed or ended for lack of the help they needed, but were denied. The VA does keep us on pills that mask our emotions. Many of us walk around like zombies – with no real life to live. I've shared with you the shame I carry every day for surviving when so many of my brothers and sisters did not. I am grateful that their deaths were not due to a conscious decision I made. Yet the VA, by making the conscious decision not to give the vets the help they so desperately need, is sentencing too many of them to lives of despair or worse. I wonder… where is the shame for that?

This is the story of hundreds if not thousands of veterans, male and female. Some vets saw more "action" and some less. Some have PTSD without going to war. Yet the government does not want to admit to these problems, for a variety of reasons. The Department of Veterans Affairs is under the Department of Defense, which seems to be of the opinion that what is not good for the current defense of the country is not worth the time or expense of the government.

I believe that the Department of Defense and the VA fear that if they become public about trauma related problems, others will not volunteer to serve our country. But I think Americans are made of stronger stuff, and I sincerely believe that most would be willing to serve their country anyway. At least this is my hope.

If only the country would begin to acknowledge that service, my hope would be even greater.

CONCLUSION

This is the conclusion of this book, but "Conclusion" only refers to the fact that you now know me, my secrets, and the life I have lived and am living. I hope that my story will have an impact on victims and the public alike. For victims, I hope that my story will give you hope. For the public, I hope there is now a better understanding that the wars of our country are not over just because the president declares them over. Some live the battles for the rest of their lives.

I also hope that the public does not forget that PTSD strikes many others besides those who have served in combat. Police officers and firefighters are particularly prone to PTSD because of the nature of their jobs. Rape victims, male and female, often have it as well. Many sources of trauma can end up destroying the lives of the victims, and all of these victims are much like the veterans I know.

Veterans are a lost sub-set of our culture. Those who cannot return as normal, productive members of society become invisible: we walk by them every day in the street, and most of us do not see them. The "hermits" who lurk deep in the woods of upper Minnesota, or in the mountains throughout the country, are routinely written off as being mentally ill. To make the situation worse, funding for the quality care of veterans is drying up. I am part of a generation that has often been referred to as "crazy Vietnam veterans." But PTSD is hardly confined to my generation or to "my" war. It has occurred in all wars and will continue with our troops in Iraq, and those in the next war, and the next.

Most of society does not really want to know the real cost of freedom; this is something that is easier forgotten. Many Americans, tired of hearing all the bad news from Iraq, are not really feeling anything for the troops that are still there and still dying. Most people go through their lives working their way up the corporate ladder, raising their families, and acquiring their riches. They take so much for granted. Travel in our country is free. We are not watched by secret police and – at least for the time being – we have protection of rights that most countries in the world can only dream of attaining. Only a small portion of our society has experienced the real *cost* of freedom.

What most Americans experience is a sanitized version of the realities of war, from "embedded" and controlled news sources. The images we see in the media are images that present a picture of the "glories" of battle, instead of the true sights and sounds of war. We are truly blessed in this country that so many can live their lives without any major traumas. The downside is that they really do not want to hear about those who are less fortunate, nor do they feel any obligation to those who have risked everything to allow them their freedoms. So many speak of patriotism, but patriotism does not stop at flag raising and fireworks. It must continue as an outstretched, helping hand for those who are left with fewer options in life as a result of their willingness to fight for this great county.

During the Iraq war, there were banners everywhere that stated "We Support Our Troops." Once the president said the war was over, these banners disappeared faster than Christmas lights. A few remained, but most found their way to landfills. "Support of the troops" was no longer necessary in the public's mind, no longer in vogue.

What is easy to forget are the wounded still lying in hospital beds. Some of these soldiers will heal physically, but some will forever be maimed. Some will never leave hospitals. Then there are those who seem physically healthy, but whose minds are consumed with the resounding horrors of a war from which they can never return. The evidence of their wounds might manifest immediately, or may stay stuffed deep down for decades. In any event, these brave young people gave up much of their lives for their country. They may not be a part of the lists of dead soldiers, but often wish they were. Dreams have been shattered, potentials have evaporated, and they are not the same as when they left. And to add insult to grievous injury, the best advice most people seem to have for them is to "get over it."

It is not that easy — and often it is not possible.

Most can never go home again. But it's damn well time we do something – anything we can – to try to bring them home anyway. They did their duty. Now it is time for the rest of us to do ours.

ABOUT THE AUTHOR

Greg Helle lives in Ankeny, Iowa. A lifelong Iowa resident, he grew up on a small farm outside Dakota City. He is married to his high school sweetheart, Alice, with whom he has just celebrated 33 years of marriage. Greg has two grown children. His daughter Lorna is a police officer in Des Moines, Iowa. His son Sean is in his third year of law school at the University of Iowa. Both children are now married. Greg was a CPA (retired status now), currently on total disability from his job and the Department of Veterans Affairs.

For Greg, PTSD is a daily struggle, the only help being those times when he is in remission through medications and therapy. However, it is much better now than it has been over the last six years. There is no cure, but he continues to hope for a good life and hopes to be enjoying grandchildren someday soon.

This is the second book Greg has written about post traumatic stress disorder. His first book is his poetic journal that he kept while going through treatment. The book is entitled "A Walk in Hell...The Other Side of War", and it can be found on his web site (www.ptsd-alliance.org/AWALKINHELL.htm). It is also available from other online bookstores. Greg has also written a play called "Tiger Cage" which is about his first visit to the Vietnam War Memorial.

Greg has also founded a non-profit corporation called PTSD Alliance. This organization is a dream of Greg's since he wants to be an advocate for trauma victims and wants to develop a way for victims to talk to other victims. Many victims are more likely to talk to another victim before they will talk with and trust professionals. Ultimately, Greg's journey – and thus, this book – is about trust. For too many American veterans, that trust has been shattered by their experiences and betrayed by their country. It is the author's hope that, in some small way, his efforts will help in the rebuilding of that trust, and the reclaiming of lives lost or discarded. To all his brothers and sisters, he bids a fond…

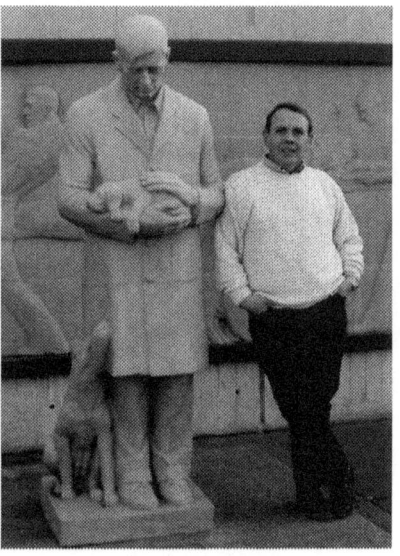

"Welcome Home."

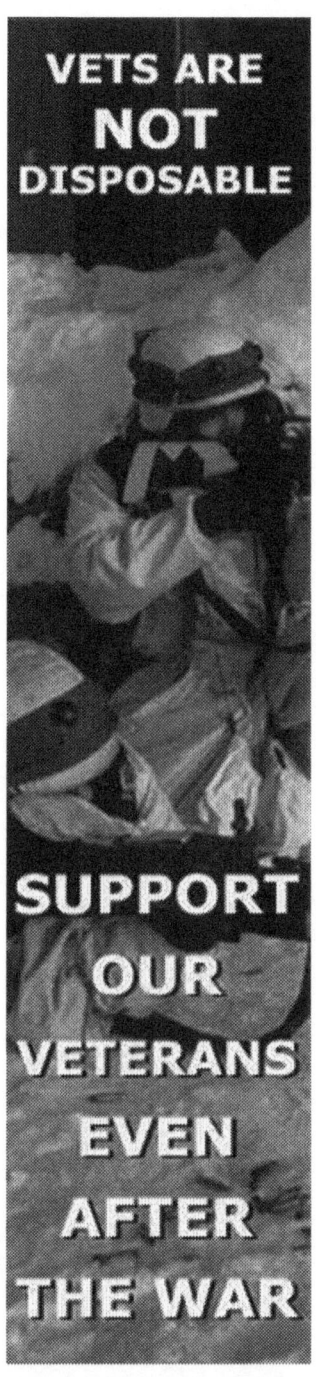

VETS ARE
NOT
DISPOSABLE

SUPPORT
OUR
VETERANS
EVEN
AFTER
THE WAR

www.ptsd-alliance.org

www.ingramcontent.com/pod-product-compliance
Lightning Source LLC
Chambersburg PA
CBHW030319290526
45785CB00001B/424